Epilepsy

Graham Scambler

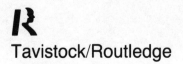

Tavistock/Routledge

For

Annette, Nikki, Sasha,
Rebecca and Miranda

First published in 1989 by
Routledge
11 New Fetter Lane, London EC4P 4EE

© 1989 Graham Scambler

Phototypeset by Input Typesetting Ltd. London
Printed and bound in Great Britain by
Biddles Ltd. Guildford and King's Lynn

British Library Cataloguing in Publication Data

Scambler, Graham
Epilepsy – (The experience of illness).
1. Man. Epilepsy. Personal adjustment
I. Title   II. Series
362.1'96853

ISBN 0–415–01757–2
ISBN 0–415–01758–0 (pbk)

Contents

Tables and figures

Acknowledgements

The genesis of this book owes much to others. Anthony Hopkins initiated the community study of adults with epilepsy which introduced me to the area. It is to him that I owe much of my knowledge and interest in epilepsy. I am also indebted to the people with epilepsy who consented to be interviewed and whose comments have been drawn on extensively throughout the book. George Brown patiently supervised a Ph.D. thesis which grew out of the community study, offering wise counsel along the way. Without Annette Scambler's support neither the study nor this text would have been completed. Finally, the editors of this series of volumes, Ray Fitzpatrick and Stanton Newman, offered detailed and constructive advice on a draft manuscript, which I appreciated and tried to heed. I retain responsibility, of course, for the final product.

Editors' preface

Epilepsy has often been considered a disorder surrounded by myths and misconceptions. For the individual who experiences epilepsy popular beliefs can constitute as great a source of difficulties as those posed by the symptoms of the disorder. Whilst medicine has made great strides in the diagnosis and management of epilepsy, the social and psychological consequences for the individual have until recently been neglected.

Graham Scambler has conducted a number of studies in this field. He has examined not only the perspectives of individuals with epilepsy and those of their families, but also popular conceptions of the disorder. In this book he brings together his many insights to provide an illuminating account of the social reality of epilepsy. In particular he critically examines one of the concepts which has been most frequently invoked to explain the social consequences of epilepsy: stigma. He develops a subtle and sensitive understanding of the diverse ways in which individuals come to sense a social disadvantage arising from the diagnosis of epilepsy. Patients' accounts are used to portray the different stages of the experience of epilepsy, from the onset of symptoms through the process of diagnosis to long-term adjustment. In so doing, he demonstrates the distinctive contribution that the social sciences can play in understanding illness.

Chapter one

The medical conception of epilepsy

Much of this volume focuses on the concept of epilepsy used within contemporary medicine. But it is appropriate to acknowledge at the outset that this concept belongs to a specific time and milieu. Not only have physicians in the past used the word epilepsy to stand for a wide range of essentially different concepts, but lay persons – including those suffering from epilepsy themselves – continue to use it in ways doctors would neither recognize nor approve. There is, then, no *one* concept of epilepsy (indeed, even within medicine nosological controversies surrounding epilepsy persist). Although it tends to be glossed over in the medical literature, this is an important point and one to which we shall regularly return.

Defining epilepsy medically: some basic concepts

There is a reasonable consensus in neurological medicine as to how epilepsy should be defined. Importantly, it is a symptom rather than a disease. An epileptic seizure is the product of an abnormal paroxysmal discharge of cerebral neurones, and epilepsy itself is sometimes defined as a continuing tendency to epileptic seizures. The use of the word 'continuing' is designed to exclude, for example, the case of the person who has a single seizure at the age of 20 and none thereafter. Such a person may be said to have experienced an epileptic seizure but not to be suffering from epilepsy. Doctors sometimes vary, however, on what constitutes 'a continuing tendency to epileptic seizures'. What if the person already referred to has a second seizure at the age of 50? Can he or she be said to have epilepsy from this point on? Or should the diagnosis be backdated thirty years? Consider also the person who had a series of seizures in adolescence but none after the age of 21. When can he or she be said to have ceased to suffer from epilepsy? After five years free from seizures? Or ten years? Or is epilepsy a lifetime diagnosis?

Epileptic seizures may take a number of different forms, depending on the site of the abnormal neuronal discharge in the brain. If the discharge remains confined to one part of the brain, the resultant seizure is described as a *partial seizure*. What happens during a partial seizure is contingent upon the exact site and pattern of discharge of abnormal neurones. If the abnormal discharge begins in one part of the brain but subsequently spreads to all parts (i.e. through the involvement of the mesodiencephalic system), the seizure is said to be a *partial seizure with secondary generalization*. Sometimes the abnormal discharge originates in the mesodiencephalic system and spreads more or less simultaneously to all parts of the brain. Such a seizure, generalized at onset, is known as a *primary generalized seizure*.

It may be helpful at this stage to describe some of the more common forms of seizure in detail. *Grand mal* seizures are a type of generalized seizure. With some *grand mal* seizures the abnormal neuronal discharge originates in the mesodiencephalic system and is generalized from the start, probably reaching all parts of the cortex simultaneously. With others the seizure results from a discharge arising from a focal lesion and spreading widely to involve the mesodiencephalic system; in this case there may be a brief warning or 'aura'. As the discharge is generalized the person is struck unconscious and falls rigidly to the ground. This is the tonic phase, characterized by powerful muscular contraction; air is forced from the chest through the larynx, sometimes resulting in a 'cry', and the teeth are clenched. No respiratory movements occur and the person rapidly becomes cyanosed. The tonic phase lasts for about half a minute and is followed by the clonic phase, consisting of violent convulsive movements of the limbs which occur at a gradually decreasing frequency. The lips and tongue may be bitten. The combination of relaxed sphincters and the contraction of the abdominal musculature may cause incontinence of urine and, less often, faeces. The clonic phase lasts for, on average, 2–3 minutes, and is followed by a complete relaxation of the muscles; the person lies still, normal ventilation returning. The period of unconsciousness generally lasts for a few minutes.

On recovering consciousness the person is likely to be confused, usually for 20 minutes to an hour, and may complain of headaches, nausea or drowsiness.

With *petit mal* seizures, which are largely seizures of childhood, all the cortical neurones are again affected more or less simultaneously. *Petit mal* consists of brief interruptions of consciousness: sudden arrest of movement and speech occurs and the person may appear pale and his or her eyelids flutter. The person does not fall down and is frequently unaware that anything has happened; to an observer he or she may seem dazed or to be daydreaming. The seizures are short-lived, lasting only a few seconds, and recovery is immediate; there are no sequelae. Whereas a person would be unfortunate to have more than one *grand mal* seizure in a day, *petit mal* seizures may occur much more frequently, ten to fifty a day being occasionally encountered.

As already noted, partial or focal seizures begin in and remain confined to neurones in the proximity of an area of local cerebral damage; this damage may be due, for example, to birth injury. The clinical symptomatology depends on the site of the damage. One common site is the *temporal lobe* and, as this portion of the brain is concerned with complex higher cortical functions, the resulting symptomatology may be complex. The person may experience hallucinations of sight, sound, taste, smell, touch, and memory. These hallucinations may be of simple sensory phenomena such as odours or single sounds, or may consist of highly developed psychic disturbances. The person often has difficulty in identifying the sensory experience. The gustatory and olfactory hallucinations tend to be unpleasant and may be accompanied by chewing movements and smacking of the lips. Hallucinatory voices and visions are not uncommon. The actual experience may be frightening or may make the person feel disquieted for no obvious reason; rarely, it gives rise to a sense of ecstasy. Two transient disturbances of memory are common: *déjà vu* (an undue sense of familiarity with an unfamiliar environment) and *jamais vu* (a feeling of unfamiliarity with a known environment). During the seizure the person does not fall unconscious but remains in a dreamy state for a few seconds to minutes. Questions may be answered in a confused manner, or the person may subsequently state that although he or she was able to comprehend what was said during the seizure it was not possible to reply. Coordinated behaviour may continue throughout (for example, dressing), or, alternatively, there may be stereotyped movements, often involving the jaw and facial muscles.

Several hundred other forms of epileptic seizure have been recorded (see the 'Commission on Classification and Terminology of the International League Against Epilepsy', 1981). Table 1.1, adapted from the WHO International Classification of Epilepsy, gives an indication of the complexity of current classificatory schemes.

Table 1.1 Adaptation of the WHO International Classification of Epilepsy

1 *Generalized Seizures*
Bilateral symmetrical seizures without local onset; clinically:
(a) Absences (*petit mal*)
(b) Bilateral myoclonus
(c) Infantile spasms
(d) Clonic seizures
(e) Tonic seizures
(f) Tonic–clonic seizures (*grand mal*)
(g) Akinetic seizures

2 *Partial Seizures*
Seizures beginning locally with:
(a) Elementary symptomatology
motor
sensory
autonomic
(b) Complex symptomatology
impaired consciousness
complex hallucinations
affective symptoms
automatism
(c) Partial seizures becoming generalized tonic–clonic seizures

3 *Unclassified Seizures*
Seizures which cannot be classified because of incomplete data

Source: World Health Organization

What is the relation between forms of seizure and types of epilepsy? Since it is generally understood that all partial seizures arise from some focal area of structural abnormality in the brain, all partial seizures, plus those seizures which are secondarily generalized from some focal onset, can be described as symptomatic of an underlying problem: *symptomatic epilepsy*. Primary generalized epilepsy is never symptomatic of underlying structural brain damage, and can be described as constitutional or *idiopathic epilepsy*.

Causes of epilepsy

The causes of epilepsy are as complex as their manifestations. *Genetic* factors are undoubtedly important, although less so than was assumed a generation ago. They are important in a number of different ways. Some rare genetic disorders can lead to epilepsy. In some of these the relevant gene is recessive; in other words, its effects are only felt if a child inherits one relevant gene from each parent (the parents each carry the gene but, as the other member of the gene pair is normal, are themselves symptomless carriers). Disorders of the brain metabolism known as lipidoses (for example, Tay–Sachs disease) come into this category. In other genetically determined disorders inheritance is through a dominant gene; one parent carrying the relevant gene shows the effects him or herself and also transmits it to, on average, half his or her children. The remaining children receive the other member of the relevant gene pair. Tuberose sclerosis and neurofibromatosis are examples here.

There is evidence that primary generalized idiopathic epilepsy may also be inherited. The biochemical abnormality which causes the abnormal EEG characteristic of this type of epilepsy appears to be inherited, although this abnormality is not invariably associated with clinical seizures. It has been suggested that the biochemical abnormality is transmitted as a dominant gene. Research indicates that about one-third of the children to whom it is transmitted – that is, one-third of half of all the children of the relationship (i.e. one-sixth) – will have seizures, although this may amount to no more than a few *petit mal* seizures in childhood. The fact that the inherited biochemical abnormality is not invariably associated with seizures accounts for the presence of primary generalized epilepsy in children whose parents have never experienced clinical seizures themselves.

It seems that a low convulsive threshold may be inherited. Thus, for example, people who develop epilepsy after a severe head injury are slightly more likely to have a family history of epilepsy than are those who do not develop epilepsy after a comparable injury. There is also a genetic component to the tendency to febrile convulsions. A febrile convulsion, if protracted, may lead to damage to one of the brain's temporal lobes. The resultant scar in the temporal lobe may then be a focus from which paroxysmal discharges (seizures) spread in later childhood or adulthood.

Congenital malformations, present at birth but not inherited, provide another cause of epilepsy. The abnormality most relevant here is a maldevelopment of blood vessels, an angioma, which results in neighbouring neurones being starved of oxygen, thus forming a seizure focus. *Anoxia*, or reduction of oxygen reaching the brain, may occur at birth, in febrile convulsions or following stroke. In each case neurones die or are damaged in such a way that they may paroxysmally discharge subsequently. Neurones may also be damaged as a consequence of physical *trauma*, either at birth or later, due for example to head injury from a road accident. Intracranial surgery is an additional source of trauma associated with subsequent epilepsy.

Brain *tumours* may cause epilepsy, almost certainly by damaging neighbouring neurones. Most primary brain tumours arise either in the glia, the supporting cells between neurones, or in the meninges, the brain's covering membranes; these tumours are termed gliomas and meningiomas respectively. For different reasons both are difficult to remove surgically.

Certain *infectious diseases* can cause epilepsy. Bacterial meningitis can lead at any age to damaged cortical cells which may subsequently act as seizure foci. Viral meningitis is a self-limiting condition which does not cause epilepsy. However, sometimes viruses do not remain confined to the brain's surface but penetrate within: this is known as encephalitis, and seizures may follow. Bacterial brain abscesses and a number of parasites can also cause epileptic seizures.

Epilepsy can also be caused by *acquired metabolic diseases*. Hypoglycaemia (low blood glucose concentration) and hypocalcaemia (low serum calcium) can both lead to seizures in the newborn. And in adulthood other acquired metabolic disease, like chronic renal failure, can cause seizures.

Not only can *alcohol* precipitate seizures but chronic alcoholism can result in the loss of cerebral neurones and hence epilepsy. Finally, some *degenerative disorders* (for example, Alzheimer's disease or pre-senile dementia) are associated with epilepsy.

It is not always possible to identify a cause for epilepsy with any confidence. In fact, several studies suggest there may be no discernible cause for the seizures of 40–70 per cent of all sufferers, although this may partly be a function of under-investigation. If the term 'cause' refers to 'more or less steady-state background factors such as the scarring of a brain following meningitis', the term 'precipitation' refers to 'short term stimuli such as exposure to television sets in susceptible people' (Hopkins 1987: 115). Table 1.2 lists some of the more common suggested precipitants of seizures. However, it is not always easy in practice to distinguish between 'cause' and 'precipitant', as Hopkins illustrates with a hypothetical case:

Take a man with a moderate genetic predisposition to seizures. Add the effects of a moderate cranial injury some two years before. Add also the effects of 'stress' at the office during the preceding month. Add also the effects of amitriptyline prescribed to help with the depression associated with this stress. If this man then has a seizure after consuming a moderate amount of alcohol the night before, what caused it – the genetic propensity, the cranial injury, the stress, the alcohol and associated metabolic changes, the disturbance of sleep associated with the depression, or the amitriptyline? Depending upon the perspective of the world of both patient and neurologist, agreement may be reached to blame just one of all these factors, quite illogically.

(Hopkins 1987: 124–5)

Table 1.2 Common suggested precipitants of seizures

Sleep	Reflex causes
Waking	glare, flashing lights, television
Deprivation of sleep	reading
Menstrual cycle	sounds
Toxic and metabolic causes	thinking
Acute alcohol intoxication	startle
Withdrawal from alcohol	movement
Drugs	Stressful life events
Hypoglycaemia	
Hypoxia	

Source: Hopkins 1987

Investigating and treating epilepsy

A number of medical investigations are used to complement the accounts of seizures of people with epilepsy themselves or their relatives. These may serve to consolidate the diagnosis, help determine seizure type, or inform theories of causation. The most common form of investigation is electroencephalography (EEG).

Electrodes with sensitive leads are attached to the scalp and the electrical activity from each lead recorded on a graph. These recordings take the form of 'waves', the height of which is determined by the voltage of the underlying activity. Each wave occurs with varying frequency, and various combinations of frequencies and voltage types can be discerned. For example, a 3-per-second spike and wave discharge synchronus in both hemispheres is characteristic of *petit mal*; this pattern accompanies seizures and can often be observed between them.

While the EEG can throw light on the type and area of origin of some epileptic seizures, its usefulness should not be exaggerated. First, it is rare for actual seizures to be recorded. Thus its usefulness is largely dependent on interseizure abnormalities (although the likelihood of detecting such abnormalities can be enhanced by various activation techniques: for example, hyperventilation, photic stimulation, sleep recording with barbiturates). Second, EEG reporting remains to some extent subjective, reports on the same trace occasionally varying from one reporter to another. Sutherland and his colleagues conclude:

Sometimes patients are incorrectly diagnosed as 'epileptic' on the basis of an ill-defined history of a turn and an EEG report 'consistent with epilepsy' while others are incorrectly regarded as normal when there is a similar history and a normal EEG report. The EEG at times can be markedly misleading.
(Sutherland *et al*. 1974: 72)

Long-term EEG monitoring in epilepsy may hold more promise but remains technically difficult and is as yet rarely considered in Britain.

The EEG is a measure of cerebral function. The optimum technique for studying cerebral structure is computed axial tomography (CAT or CT scanning). CT scanning may give a visual demonstration of a structural abnormality causing seizures. Interestingly, the increasingly routine use of this potent technique has lent conviction to the view that idiopathic epilepsy is somewhat rarer than it was thought to be, and that minor structural abnormalities, undetected by earlier and cruder investigations, may prove to be the cause of most instances of epilepsy. Some investigations have been largely superseded by CT scanning (for example, air encephalography), but a number of others remain useful. Arteriography may be helpful in relation to people with a tumour or angioma for whom surgery is a possibility. Lumbar punctures are conducted when individuals develop seizures in the presence of an acute neurological disorder like meningitis. Biopsies of the skin abnormalities associated with tuberose sclerosis or neurofibromatosis may confirm a suspected diagnosis. Simple blood tests and skull X-rays are cheap and sometimes useful options which continue to be widely deployed.

The main form of treatment for epilepsy is drugs. The majority of people can be rendered seizure-free by pharmacological means, although chronic intractable epilepsy develops in approximately 20 per cent of cases. Occasionally surgery may be appropriate for those who have a single discrete focal abnormality and whose seizures have been unresponsive to drug therapy, but the proportion of those with epilepsy likely to benefit from surgery will probably remain small. Sometimes people can learn to control their seizures by avoiding clear precipitants, for example alcohol or lack of sleep. But the large majority require anti-convulsant medication, often over a period of many years.

Five drugs are commonly used for the management of partial and *grand mal* seizures: phenytoin, carbamazepine, sodium valporate, phenobarbitone and primidone. All show similar therapeutic results, but phenobarbitone and primidone tend to be used less because of their sedative effects.

All these drugs, however, have important toxic effects, both on the central nervous system and other tissues, and often the dose chosen for a particular patient is a balance between adequate control of seizures and avoidance of toxicity. Behavioural disturbance and impairment of learning are possible problems, particularly in children. Carbamazepine is often recommended for partial (focal) seizures, sodium valporate for tonic–clonic (grand mal) seizures, and phenytoin for both types, but recent clinical trials suggest that there is little difference between the anti-epileptic effect of the three drugs in these types of epilepsy, although tonic–clonic seizures respond to them better than partial seizures.

(DHSS 1986: 14)

Petit mal seizures are generally treated with either sodium valporate or ethosuximide, the advantage of the former being that it is also effective against co-existent *grand mal* seizures.

Occasionally, one seizure may follow another without full recovery between them; this is known as *status epilepticus*. Status epilepticus with *grand mal* seizures is a medical emergency. The lack of normal respiratory movements, in association with the extreme muscular contractions during the seizures, throw considerable stress on the cardiovascular system. And the prolonged lack of oxygen can lead to brain damage. Benzodiazepine drugs like diazepine and clonazepine are the drugs of choice in these fairly rare circumstances.

Epidemiological aspects of epilepsy

Nothing has yet been written about the numbers of people suffering from epilepsy. This is because it was necessary to indicate the complexity of epileptic phenomena before issues of incidence and prevalence could be meaningfully raised. There are two major problems in the collection of statistics about epilepsy. The first concerns case ascertainment. Most studies have been hospital-based, and it is clear that any sample of people with epilepsy derived exclusively from hospital sources will reflect any bias in selection of the hospital. Thus people with inactive or untreated epilepsy have been under-represented in these studies. Many community-based studies, however, have been brief audits, and even in the more extensive surveys case selection has rarely been comprehensive. The second problem concerns diagnostic criteria. In community studies especially the criteria for inclusion have been highly variable and, in some instances, unspecified in published reports.

Incidence is the rate at which new cases of a disorder occur, and for epilepsy the average annual incidence is usually calculated per 100,000. Zielinsky (1982) has argued that since the estimate of new cases is based on the number of first cases of epilepsy diagnosed, the rate would be more appropriately termed 'accession rate'. There may be a gap of some years between the first seizure and the diagnosis of epilepsy. And there are those who never consult a doctor or whose condition is never diagnosed. Hence the accession rate may fall considerably below the real rate. Most studies give annual incidence rates of 20–25 per 100,000. The rates are highest in the pre-school years (especially the first year of life), fall rapidly in the second decade, and remain low at least until the age of 60. Many studies show continuing low rates for people over 60. However, there are exceptions: one of the most impressive epidemiological analyses of epilepsy, carried out in Rochester, Minnesota, from the Mayo Clinic, shows a considerable increase in the rates for people aged 60 and above (Hauser and Kurland 1975).

Prevalence refers to the frequency of current cases of a disorder, and for epilepsy is generally estimated per 1,000. Estimates of the prevalence of active epilepsy – that is, those who have had two or more non-febrile seizures and have either had a seizure within the previous two years or are on anticonvulsant medication – usually range from 3–6 per 1,000. Table 1.3 gives the distribution of types of seizure from one British community study (Hopkins and Scambler 1977). Most studies show a slight excess of males with epilepsy and higher rates in the lower socio-economic groups. Most studies also show the lowest rates of epilepsy for the first decade of life, an increase thereafter, and a falling off after the age of 50. The Rochester study is again exceptional in reporting high rates in older age groups; this may be the result of more effective methods of case identification showing up the accumulation of cases.

Table 1.3 Distribution of different types of seizure in the community (%)

Seizures experienced	Typical absences	Partial seizure	Tonic–clonic	Seizure of any of these three types
In past 2 months	2	37	26	50
In past 2 years	2	45	47	69
At any time	7	56	95	100

Source: Hopkins and Scambler 1977

In addition to the 56% who had experienced a partial seizure at some time, there was clear clinical or EEG evidence of partial onset to generalized seizures in a further 12%.
(n = 94)

Studies of prognosis of people with epilepsy have tended to focus on the issues of remission of symptoms and survival (Schoenberg 1985). Hauser *et al.* (1982) studied seizure recurrence after a first unprovoked seizure among patients presenting at four large hospitals in Minneapolis–St. Paul in the US. The cumulative risk of a subsequent seizure was 27 per cent at three years after the initial episode, the risk of recurrence being greatest in those who had suffered a prior neurological insult. Findings like this help account for the reluctance of most researchers to include single, isolated seizures in the definition of epilepsy. In a recent community-based study of prognosis in Britain, however, seizures recurred in as many as four out of five patients after the first seizure (Goodridge and Shorvon 1983). Although the authors add that this may be an overestimate, since some individuals with single seizures may have been overlooked or have concealed them, it does suggest that recurrence may be more common than has been supposed.

Using available data on prevalence and incidence, Hauser (1978) has estimated that the average duration of symptoms among people with epilepsy is about 12 years. Hauser and Kurland (1975) found that the percentage of patients who had been seizure-free for at least 2 years at the latest follow-up was 40 per cent at 10 years after the initial diagnosis, 49 per cent at 15 years, and 55 per cent at 20 years. At 20 years 40 per cent had been free from seizures for 10 years or more. Goodridge and Shorvon found a similar if more pronounced falling-off of seizures. They emphasize the importance of what they term the 'temporal aspects of prognosis':

> We found that most patients entered remission early, the longer the epilepsy remained active the less likely was eventual remission, and relapse after remission was relatively rare. It follows that the long term prognosis for epilepsy in this population could have been predicted from its early course. At an arbitrary point of five years after the first seizure, for instance, of those whose epilepsy was still active, only 21 per cent achieved subsequent terminal remission compared with 96 per cent of those who were already in remission.
>
> (Goodridge and Shorvon 1983: 647)

Recalling Gowers' view over a century ago that 'each fit facilitates the occurrence of the next', they continue: 'Most patients who developed epilepsy were treated, and their condition then took a well circumscribed, short-lived course, which suggests that treatment might be "curative" ' (1983: 647).

Survival data among individuals with epilepsy are also forthcoming from the Rochester studies. The observed survival of all people identified as suffering from epilepsy in the Rochester population was compared to expected survival, based on the experience of an age- and sex-matched comparison group from the same area. Relative survival – observed/expected – was 91 per cent at five years after diagnosis, and 85 per cent at both 10 and 15 years. Those whose seizures were due to a recognized primary disorder, such as a brain tumour, and those whose seizures began before the age of five had the poorest prognosis in relation to survival.

Chapter two

Becoming a patient: aspects of care

What is often lacking in textbook descriptions of epileptic seizures is any real indication of what it is like to experience them. This chapter opens with a brief consideration of sufferers' own accounts of their seizures. The discussion then focuses on people's conceptualizations and responses to their *first* epileptic episode; on the decision to consult a physician; on the physician's diagnosis of epilepsy and the reactions this can elicit; and on aspects of people's careers as patients and of continuing management and care.

Experiencing seizures

For some individuals with epileptic seizures the question 'What do they feel like?' has little significance. This is because they have neither warnings that seizures are about to occur nor awareness of the seizures when they do: 'I'm like in another world. I don't know what's happened!' And not all those who are conscious of having seizures (i.e. those with partial seizures or with generalized seizures resulting from a discharge arising from a focal lesion and preceded by an aura) are able to translate their experiences into words: 'It's something you really can't explain. You've got to, sort of, experience it!'

Accounts of seizures which are volunteered indicate something of the variety of sensations experienced and their occasionally frightening or disturbing nature (Scambler 1983):

> The funny thing is you know when you're going to have it, but you don't actually know when you have it. . . . It's an awful feeling, you know: you feel as though you want to talk to somebody and you can't.

You get a warning, then panic sets in because you know what's going to happen. . . . It seems to take a long time, but obviously it's only a few seconds. But they're the worst seconds, when you know you're going to go and there's nothing you can do.

A tremendous noise used to build up in the ears, what they call an aura. It used to build up to a colossal pitch: it was like a bell ringing, but it was, how can I say . . . it was ringing at a wrong tone. And then that was it: you knew no more after that.

I can see myself now, sitting in that chair, and your mouth opens and you, you let out such a bawl, trying to tell somebody. But you can't speak: its impossible!

I used to get a peculiar taste in my mouth and a sort of ringing in the ears . . . and I used to feel weak; and then I'd fall down. I didn't shake. I didn't appear to be having a fit. I just appeared to pass out, although I never lost consciousness.

Well, I know I'm going to get one, just a few seconds before, and I sit down. I gulp, I can feel myself swallowing all the time; and the first thing I think is: 'Where am I? What day is it?' and 'What am I doing here?' And although I'm going through this funny thing, I'm aware of it. I think: 'Oh no, I've got one of these things coming on me!' And then, all of a sudden, I snap out of it and I feel tired and drowsy.

A lot of them have involved, have sort of happened while I've been talking to people . . . and I tend to get mesmerized. I sort of don't listen to what they're saying; I just watch the action of their lips. It's a bit like hypnosis in a sense – most peculiar.

I had this numbness in my left arm and side: it was almost like a stroke – even my face was, sort of, half-dropped. It was a most peculiar thing. And I could feel this twitching, like an electric shock, in my left arm, and then I lost consciousness.

Well, all I know is, I come over a bit sweaty, then I start – it's like a cough; and then all of a sudden my hands start getting tight, but there's no feeling in them, they're numb; but I know – I can see them – they're shaking.

You know you're not able to cope with whoever's talking to you. And yet you still look normal, you know? You don't look ill, so they'll get you a drink of water; you just look the same. And if they're waiting for an answer, you know they are, and you can't think to speak. I always used to say: 'I'll try and have a line ready that I could say each time, like: "Excuse me, I don't feel well".' But it never, ever happens that you do it. It's a horrible feeling, because people are looking at you and you can feel them waiting . . . I mean it must look terribly stupid to someone . . . You work yourself up to a pitch in those few seconds, trying to make your brain work. You never can but you do it automatically.

Aware of their seizures or not, nine out of every ten in the study from which these quotations are drawn recalled feeling anxious or upset about their possible consequences. Most often mentioned was the fact that seizures could be stigmatizing:

It's rather humiliating actually, sort of 'coming to' on a London Underground station – and, you know, the whole train's stopped because of you, and you've been carried onto the platform, and you've got soaking wet trousers. . . . It's a terrible feeling when it happens in public like that.

I was embarrassed in front of a lot of people, you know, a lot of my friends. I hoped none of them had seen through it, you know, realized what it was.

Seizures also commonly caused anxiety through their capacity to disrupt normal activities: 'I don't go out much in case I have one in the streets, get picked up, and taken to hospital'. Some brought incidental injury:

The most upsetting attack I had was when I lost my teeth, and I was lucky I wasn't blinded. . . . I should have stayed in the chair, but I came over all bad . . . I was going to the street door to get a bit of air . . . I had a blackout and fell on the chair. My chin went on the chair and it loosened these teeth; but I was lucky because the shock, the impact, it sort of sent my glasses flying. I was scared stiff because I might have been blinded.

And others dashed hopes of remissions or recovery: 'I'm on a time trial. I'm sort of going for a record: I'm trying not to have one for as long as possible. So when I have one, it's ruined 18 months or a year, sort of thing! I've got to start again.' An added source of worry was that both seizures and their sequelae can bring unhappiness in equal measure to others, especially family members.

The first episode

It is apparent from these comments that people's responses to their seizures are often related to the contexts in which they occur. In Scambler and Hopkins' community survey of adults with epilepsy, approximately a quarter of those interviewed defined the first seizure they had experienced – often whilst in childhood – as the most upsetting *because it was the first* (Scambler 1983). Thus, 'the first, I think, was the most frightening really, because it just came, literally, out of the blue.' From the accounts they gave, most people were distressed for one of three reasons. First, the seizure was itself sometimes disturbing: some people were aware that something new, strange and irresistible was happening to them. This was generally disconcerting and may have been the lot of as many as one in three of the sample. Mr R. was 32 years old at onset:

> I started stuttering. I was rather concerned about it because I couldn't seem to control it. I went indoors and upstairs to an old friend. I was sitting on a chair talking to him, and I went to say a particular word – I can't remember the word now – and it just stuck, and I stuttered, and it went on and on; and then my head went back and I saw the look on their faces and my wife's panic. They both rushed over to me, and that was the last I remembered. . . . Apparently I had a *grand mal*, or something like this; a big fit, quite a serious fit.

Mrs G., a schoolgirl of 11 when she had her first seizure, recalled being terrified: 'The first thing I thought was: "Oh, I'm going to die!".'

Incidental injuries were a second source of distress, affecting one in ten. A few people regained consciousness to discover they had bitten their tongues during the clonic phase of a generalized seizure. Others were hurt when they lost consciousness and dropped to the ground. Mrs C., a single woman of 22 at onset, said:

> I went to the toilet and blacked out in there, and, in a very confined space, I crashed my head against the wall, so I was completely bruised all down my face. . . . I had terrific black eyes, bloodshot eyes, but I had no warning of it at all.

People like Mrs C., alone and with no awareness, and hence recollection, of the seizure, could only infer what had happened from the circumstances in which they found themselves on recovering consciousness. Mrs C. inferred, wrongly as it transpired, that she had merely fainted. She consulted her general practitioner solely because of the injuries sustained when she fell.

Third, many people – perhaps four out of five – were upset by others' reactions to the seizure. Some, like Mr R. already mentioned, were disturbed or frightened at the 'panic' induced. Some were simply embarrassed to have 'caused such a stir'. Most commonly, however, individuals were bewildered or alarmed at the action taken by witnesses. Often, especially when they had not been aware of the seizure and had not hurt themselves, this action seemed irrational and excessive. Mr T. explained that, 'I just woke up one morning and my wife said "You've just had a fit and I've called the doctor in".' His attitude was one of 'sheer disbelief': 'I couldn't have, and so forth . . . but then, of course, it dawned on me that I must have had one; it really worried me.' Mrs B. had her first seizure in bed:

> I apparently woke up with a terrific scream, and my husband said I shot up in bed: my eyes were open but couldn't see. . . . He called the doctor. Dr W., I think, came, and he thoroughly examined me from head to toe, and they managed to get some tablets into my mouth. And then, about 7 a.m., my husband woke me up, asking me if I was better. And I said to him: 'What are you talking about? There's nothing wrong with me!'

Miss G., who was 15, had her first seizure while doing a Saturday job in a hairdresser's. She recovered consciousness in hospital: 'And the manageress of the hairdresser's was sitting by the bed. I asked her what had happened, and she said: "You've had a fit." I said: "That's not possible, I couldn't have".' Unnerved at finding herself in hospital, and by this time feeling perfectly normal, Miss

G. continued to dispute the suggestion that she had had a 'fit' with the hospital staff.

Initial medical contact

The same survey was informative on people's initial contact with the medical profession. Of those who knew how this came about, 17 per cent were rushed to hospital by ambulance in what was termed a *panic* consultation; 54 per cent had a fairly *prompt* consultation – almost always within a few days – as a direct consequence of the first episode; 24 per cent consulted only after a *delay*, often doing so on experiencing a second seizure; and 5 per cent consulted only *incidentally* (i.e. a physician learned of the seizure 'by chance' while being consulted about some other matter). All the panic consultations were, by definition, with hospital physicians, while this was true of only 7 per cent of prompt and 2 per cent of delayed consultations. Three of four incidental consultations took place in hospital. All remaining consultations, two-thirds of the total, were with general practitioners (Scambler 1983).

Several factors seem to have influenced the pattern of events after onset. Of particular significance is the fact that four out of five consultations were initiated by someone other than the person experiencing the seizure. Nor was this merely a function of age at onset. One implication of this, of course, is that the distress associated with *experiencing* a first seizure was typically a less important determinant of consulting behaviour than the distress associated with *witnessing* one.

Predictably, other-initiated consultations were more likely than the self-initiated to have been panic or prompt and to have involved hospital physicians. Two other factors were relevant to the circumstances of the first consultation, regardless of whether it was other- or self-initiated. First, those whose first seizure was generalized were more likely to see a physician on the basis of that seizure alone than those whose first seizure was partial. It is reasonable to assume that this is due to the often dramatic properties of *grand mal* seizures in particular. And second, those whose first seizure occurred at home were more likely to see a general practitioner than those for whom onset occurred elsewhere. This again seems readily explicable, in terms of ease of access to the physician perceived as the most appropriate to attend illness in the home.

Learning of the diagnosis of epilepsy

Several parents in one study of the families of children with epilepsy complained that the diagnosis was disclosed 'much later in their child's career than was reasonable' (West 1979: 634). In their study of adults with epilepsy in the US, Schneider and Conrad (1983) found that only 35 per cent recalled a quick connection between a first, unanticipated seizure and learning of the medical diagnosis of epilepsy. In Scambler and Hopkins' (1988) study this proportion was considerably smaller. Of those with clear memories, only 11 per cent said they had been told as a result of their initial consultation. All of these learned the diagnosis within a day or two of onset. Nineteen per cent learned within a month; 11 per cent learned between one and six months after onset; 12 per cent learned between six months and one year; and 48 per cent said they learned of the diagnosis of epilepsy only after a year had elapsed. It may be, of course, that for some who waited more than a year the diagnosis was actually made and communicated shortly after onset, but to somebody other than the sufferer, perhaps a parent. This is suggested by the fact that the median age at onset varied from 27 for those who found out about the diagnosis within a day or two of their first seizure, to 15 for those who found out only after 12 months or more had passed. It is likely that sometimes the diagnostic label was either kept a parental secret or made no immediate impression on child sufferers.

Eight per cent remembered discovering the diagnosis from a member of the family; 36 per cent from their general practitioner; 48 per cent from a hospital physician; and 8 per cent 'impersonally' (for example, as a result of a chance sight of their hospital notes). Apart from the probable effect of age at onset (on the timing of the communication of the diagnosis), no other factors seemed to exercise any special influence.

Responses to the label

In his autobiography *A Sort of a Life*, Graham Greene recalls the following episode:

> 'Your mother tells me you are engaged to be married', Richmond [Greene's former psychoanalyst] said. 'Now about this fainting attack at *The Times*. . . .'
>
> I remembered how the specialist had questioned me about the earlier attacks of fainting in the summer stuffiness of the school chapel. Many children, I told myself, went through such a phase.
>
> 'Doctor Riddick diagnosed epilepsy', Richmond said. Epilepsy, cancer and leprosy – these are the three medical terms which rouse the greatest fear in the untutored, and at 22 one is unprepared for so final a judgement. Epilepsy, Richmond went on, could be inherited: I must consider the risk carefully before marriage, and he sought to comfort me by pointing out that Dostoievsky too had suffered from epilepsy. I couldn't think of a reply. Dostoievsky was a dead Victorian writer, not a youth without a book to his name who had pledged himself to marry. . . . 'Let me see your novel', Richmond said, meaning to be kind. 'What is the title?'
>
> '*The Episode*', I said.
>
> I left the house and began walking fast towards South Kensington, the King's Road, Oakley Street, the Albert Bridge, away from *this* episode. When I got home I wrote a letter; they had left things rather late, I said, before informing me. Poor souls, I can sympathize with them now as I read the letters which were written to them on the same day by Richmond and Dr Riddick. Dr Riddick's was frightening, even in its moderation. 'The attacks to which he is occasionally subject are, I think, epileptic; but since he has lost consciousness in three only, there is a reasonably good chance that, with suitable treatment, the condition may be arrested.' The treatment seemed to consist of good walks and Kepler's Malt Extract. Richmond's letter was more encouraging, and my mother in pencil has pathetically underlined all the optimistic phrases she could find, perhaps to comfort my father – 'quite likely to clear up completely' . . . 'no cause for alarm' – even the phrase about Dostoievsky

is trotted out and surprisingly underlined, but then follows
what I think was unfair and dangerous advice: 'We agreed
that Graham ought not to be told what is the matter in any
terms that included the word epilepsy.'

Was the diagnosis right? With the hindsight of forty years,
free from any recurrence, I don't believe it, but I believed it
then. I remember the next day standing on an Underground
platform and trying to summon up the will and the courage
to jump.'

(Greene 1972: 136–7)

Schneider and Conrad cite an equally extreme reaction to the
diagnosis. A woman's parents had hidden the diagnosis from her
for several months, during which time she continued to experience
seizures. When she found out:

I tried to commit suicide. I tried to take an overdose of the
drugs I was on. I felt like some unclean spirit had walked in
the door. I mean, I felt . . . uh, an oddball. Because nobody
would communicate to me what it was about . . . I felt a
great stigma attached to it.

(Schneider and Conrad 1983: 72)

Nobody in Scambler and Hopkins' study was driven this far.
However, if almost all were distressed by onset and its sequelae,
as many were much more so when they became acquainted with
the diagnosis of epilepsy. In only 20 per cent of cases had such a
possibility been entertained. A few, no more than one in twenty,
accepted the news with equanimity, but most of these had not
encountered the word epilepsy before: 'Quite honestly, I'd never
heard of it before, and so it didn't really bother me.' But the great
majority had come across the word and were upset and sometimes
angry and resentful that it had been judged applicable to their
symptoms: 'The very word epilepsy puts terror into you, doesn't
it?'

When the doctor suggested that this could be wrong with me,
I nearly went berserk! Epilepsy is a terrible word, I believe,
to some people; the same as cancer. People don't like to
mention these two words, do they?

In the course of his discussion of labelling theory, Rotenberg
rightly points out that 'social labelling' does not always lead to

'self-labelling'. The question therefore arises: 'What makes the label stick from the actor's perspective?' (Rotenberg 1974: 334). Of key importance in the case of people with epilepsy is the application of the label by a physician. As Schneider and Conrad put it, 'medical diagnoses are "realities" with which people so designated must contend, independently of the physiological aspects of their conditions' (1981: 213). Scambler and Hopkins (1986) found that people were upset by the diagnosis of epilepsy for two related reasons. First, they shared a more or less clearly defined awareness that a physician's diagnostic statement, whether made in their presence or to a third party in their absence, had transformed them from 'normal' persons into 'epileptics'. And a medical – and hence authoritative – diagnostic statement does indeed confer the social and legal status of epileptic. Second, they perceived this ascribed and unwanted status as a personal and social liability.

The status of epileptic was seen as a burden largely because people felt epilepsy to be a stigmatizing condition: a condition which rendered them unacceptably different from normal partici-pants in their social milieux (Goffman 1968). This feeling was rooted in their perceptions of contemporary public attitudes to epilepsy. And many started with a low and uncharitable view of lay opinions. This is reflected in Mrs C.'s response to learning of the diagnosis of epilepsy:

> I rather objected to having this label attached to my records from there on, and, it's probably dead ignorant on my part, but I objected to having this little stamp on my records labelling me as 'an epileptic' on what to me was just . . . I had fainted once, and then I fainted a year later a second time, and, as I said, I've got plenty of friends who faint occasionally but don't have this label attached to them. The general – not so much myself now, because I've found out a bit more about it – but the general public are still very ill-informed about epilepsy; I think they think there's some sort of demon going on . . . they're badly informed on epilepsy and they think you're something of a bit of a freak. I objected very much to the label originally.

Mrs C. implies that she was herself 'ill-informed' at first. Miss G., who was 15 when told of the diagnosis, spoke in similar fashion:

I know I was very upset. I cried about it, I know; because, as I say, I was prejudiced against other people who had them [i.e. seizures]. I don't really know, it's just, I thought they were a bit odd, people that had them. When I started having them myself: oh, it was such a terrible thing! I was still fairly young I suppose. I just thought it was terrible, that it was the end of the world, so to speak . . . because of this prejudice, the way I looked at other people: I naturally assumed that other people were going to start looking at me like that.

Because they felt epilepsy to be stigmatizing and recognised that entry to the status of epileptic was ultimately contingent upon a physician's diagnosis, many people did their best to *negotiate* a less intimidating diagnosis, to disavow the label 'epileptic'. Some, like Mrs C. quoted above, started immediately with the neurologist who told her she had epilepsy. She explained how he

got quite cross with me, in fact, when I objected. . . . He was quite annoyed that I should object. . . . He said: 'The time for you to look as you're looking now was the time when you had the first faint.' But of course it didn't mean anything to me then! He wasn't particularly understanding I must say!

Others set about their task of negotiating indirectly, through often protracted discussions with family or friends. Mr A. and his wife quickly convinced themselves of the falsity of the diagnosis; Mrs A. went on to recall a neighbour having a 'dizzy spell' diagnosed as a 'slight epileptic fit' at about the same time and concluded that 'The doctors seem to have a thing about epilepsy at the moment.' Yet others confined their negotiations to the privacy of their own minds. Mr W. confessed, 'I always thought at the back of my mind that it wasn't. I always termed epilepsy as, if you went into convulsions.' While a few managed to convince themselves, and perhaps their relatives and friends, that they were not 'properly epileptic', nobody in the study succeeded in converting their physicians.

Medical dissension and, more significantly, medical *uncertainty* about epileptic phenomena sometimes provided people with an incentive to contest the diagnosis. Fox (1975) has distinguished three types of uncertainty that beset physicians. The first stems from 'an incomplete and inadequate mastery of available knowledge'; the second is the product of 'gaps' in medical science;

and the third derives from these: 'the difficulty of distinguishing between, on the one hand, personal ignorance and ineptitude, and on the other hand, inadequacies in the present state of medical science'. People with epilepsy may be on the wrong end of all three, and to a degree peculiarly so due to the range and fundamental nature of the uncertainties of the second of Fox's triad of types. Consider, for example, the aetiology of epilepsy. In Hopkins and Scambler's (1977) study physicians were unable to identify a cause of seizures in nearly three-quarters of those seen. The equivalent figure in the study conducted in Rochester, Minnesota (and cited in Chapter 1) was 79 per cent (Hauser and Kurland 1975). Uncertainties about when to commence, change, and stop anticonvulsant therapy and about prognosis are equally common. Inevitably this uncertainty communicates itself to patients. Davis (1960) has distinguished usefully between 'real' and 'functional' uncertainty. The former refers to gaps in medical science of the kind sampled above; and the latter refers to the uses to which real (or feigned) uncertainty lends itself in the medical management of patients and their families. There is a considerable literature on functional uncertainty. In his own work on children suffering from paralytic poliomyelitis, for example, Davis shows how physicians sometimes feign uncertainty when faced with the prospect of passing on a particularly depressing prognosis:

Uncertainty is to some extent feigned by the doctor for the purpose of gradually – to use Goffman's very descriptive analogy – 'cooling the mark out', i.e. getting the patient ultimately to accept and put up with a state of being that is initially intolerable to him.

(Davis 1963: 67)

Accounts like Davis' are predicated on patient intolerance of uncertainty. Paradoxically however, while uncertainty troubled most people with epilepsy, they, as well as their physicians, capitalized on it. Most significantly, they often used real or feigned uncertainty as 'tools of negotiation' when trying to shake off the diagnostic label 'epileptic'. Several, for example, used the fact that no physician was able to put forward a credible aetiological theory of the seizures to justify their denial that they had epilepsy: 'If he doesn't even know what causes them, how can he know they're epileptic?'

Making sense of epilepsy

It does not follow from the fact that some individuals use medical uncertainty to try to distance themselves from a diagnosis of epilepsy that people are generally content with a piecemeal or fragmented understanding of their conditions. If a vacuum is created by medical ignorance or reticence, the inclination is to fill it. In her general study of disability Blaxter writes of individuals'

> strenuous attempts to see their medical history as a whole, to connect together everything that had happened to them in an attempt to provide a coherent story, in which effect followed cause in a rational way... . . There seemed to be a deep need for people to be able to make sense of their world.
>
> (1976: 221–2)

What Blaxter refers to as a 'strain towards rationality' will here be called *rationalization*. For people with epilepsy this process of rationalization may be especially salient. Whilst for most of the time feeling, appearing, and behaving entirely normally, they have to live not only with the label 'epileptic' but also with the ever present possibility of sudden, irresistible seizures, which may be frightening to experience as well as bizarre or dramatic to behold, and which may also bring about a total transformation of their immediate plans or circumstances and of the way they are regarded by others.

Scambler and Hopkins asked interviewees if they had questions they would like to put to a physician. Predictably, in the light of both previous studies and the fact that in only a quarter of cases had a cause of epilepsy been identified, over half the queries people had concerned aetiology. Comments like the following were typical:

> I know I've got epilepsy, but I don't know what it's all about. I don't know what causes it.

> If I could understand the cause of it, then I could put everything together . . . but no one hasn't told me what's the cause of it.

> You can ask them a lot of things, can't you? . . . But you don't seem to get the cause of it.

> I did say to him: 'Why do I get these?' . . . and I said: 'Why

is it me? Why do I have to have them?' I said this one day, and he said: 'There's so many thousands of people that have them, and there's so many different kinds.' He said: 'I just couldn't tell you.'

What's it in aid of? I've done no harm to anybody.

In this study parents and spouses were often heavily implicated in the construction of (lay) theories about epilepsy and its aetiology. Parents of young children seemed particularly influential. Carter (1947) found in the US that children's beliefs and attitudes towards their epilepsy were frequently derivatives of parental opinions. For this reason it will be helpful to make use of a classification first developed by Tavriger (1966) to accommodate parental theories about the causes of epilepsy.

Tavriger and her colleagues interviewed 118 parents of children with epilepsy between the ages of 3 and 15. Forty-three parents produced 53 'fantasies' related to 'the aetiology or sudden exacerbation of fits' (all 'probable real causes' were excluded from the analysis). In Table 2.1 Tavriger's classification of these fantasies is reproduced. 'It would appear', she wrote, 'that the anxiety engendered by epilepsy demands from some parents alleviation in the form of a theory as to its cause, no matter how illogical' (Tavriger 1966: 342). Having noted, following Ounsted (1955), that such theories are often stubbornly defended against professional scepticism or scorn, she went on to hypothesize that 'it may also be that the fantasy is an attempt to deny that the child has epilepsy, because the parents' fears of what this means have not

Table 2.1 Types of lay theories of the aetiology of epilepsy

	Tavriger's study		Scambler and Hopkins' study	
	%	(cases)	%	(cases)
1 Psychological:				
(a) Single trauma	9	(5)	7	(4)
(b) Prolonged stress	47	(25)	39	(22)
2 Physical:				
(a) Trauma	21	(11)	21	(12)
(b) Physiological or anatomical factors	17	(9)	21	(12)
3 Genetic	2	(1)	3	(2)
4 Other	4	(2)	9	(5)
Totals	100	(53)	100	(57)

been dealt with' (1966: 342). There is a measure of support for this hypothesis in West's (1979) study of families of children with epilepsy.

Scambler and Hopkins found that only two out of every five of those in whom a cause of epilepsy had been medically identified showed any awareness of this cause. None of those who did show some awareness, however, either challenged the medical account or complemented it with their own theories. Sixty per cent of those who knew of no medical theory of causation had generated their own aetiological theories: between them they volunteered fifty-seven such theories. Table 2.1 permits a comparison of these with the fantasies produced by the parents questioned by Tavriger's team. The distributions are remarkably similar. Most importantly perhaps, both point to 'prolonged stress' as the main focus of non-medical theorizing about the aetiology of epilepsy.

It was also apparent in both studies that some of those who postulated prolonged stress as a cause of their conditions did so primarily because they found the idea that their seizures had a 'physical' cause extremely threatening.

> Well, I'd like to think they were psychological. You see, when I don't have one for a long period of time I think to myself that it's psychological, so I think: 'I haven't had one for a year, so it must be psychological and not something physical, because it would keep recurring if it was something physical.'

This bias towards theories focusing on prolonged stress seemed generally due to one of two factors. First, underlying some people's thinking was the conviction, often unacknowledged, that if their seizures were the result of prolonged stress – merely a function of the pressures and hardships of life – then they could not be epileptic; in other words, theories of this type assisted negotiations towards the establishment of an alternative and more palatable diagnosis. Second, some felt that if their seizures were products of prolonged stress, then there must be hope of a cure. Tavriger writes: 'Some parents preferred to see epilepsy as "nerves", believing that alleviation of stresses would cure the illness' (1966: 342). This last statement suggests that people may not always have distinguished adequately between factors implicated in the aetiology of their conditions and factors precipitating individual seizures. When questioned directly about precipitating factors, 80 per cent listed some ninety-two factors, the most frequently cited of which were stressful situations, excitement and heat.

Mr H. was one of those who conflated the concepts of aetiological agent and precipitant of seizures. He was also one of the few who constructed theories independently of their families and of other potential lay referral networks. Aged 18 when interviewed, he had had three or four nocturnal seizures since onset at the age of 15. When asked to define epilepsy, he replied:

> Well, I would say epilepsy is – if you're working hard or you're really, you're hot in the head, if you know what I mean, you get headaches and you're working too much, your brain's too active, if you know what I mean, you, your brain just can't take no more and it just conks out for a little while.

He later added: 'I haven't done anything wrong. I haven't over-heated myself or anything like that'. These remarks are worth dwelling on briefly since they reflect both the personal anguish and what Tavriger would call the 'illogicality' of some lay theorizing about causation. It transpired that Mr H.'s statements combined the 'accepted' family theory (which centred on prolonged stress deriving largely from too much schoolwork) and his own private theory (hinted at in such phrases as 'you're hot in the head', 'your brain's too active', 'I haven't done anything wrong' and 'I haven't over-heated myself') which was that his seizures represented some kind of punishment for episodes of heavy petting with his girlfriend. Asked by his general practitioner to keep a record of his seizures, he had noticed that they correlated closely with his sexual excesses, and had concluded that his seizures reflected the wrath of some higher moral authority. His allegiance to his theory was weakening by the time of interview, however, his latest excess having apparently gone unpunished (Scambler 1983).

Aspects of the management of epilepsy

For most people with epilepsy responsibility for the management of their condition is shared by their general practitioner and one or more (usually more) hospital specialists. Figure 2.1, taken from the recent *Report of the Working Group on Services for People*

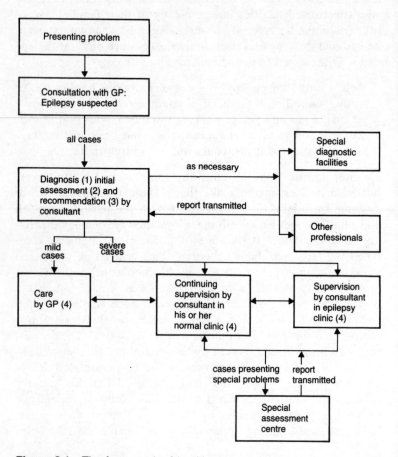

Figure 2.1 The framework of health care

Notes

(1) The diagnosis may be that the person does not have epilepsy, but for the purposes of this chart if is assumed that epilepsy is confirmed.

(2) In certain circumstances epilepsy clinics may carry out diagnosis and initial assessment.

(3) 'Recommendation' includes the possibility that no treatment is considered appropriate.

(4) The arrangements for continuing supervision will depend on whether specific problems persist, recur, or develop; patients may need to be referred between the consultant, GP, and epilepsy clinic if their condition changes.

with Epilepsy (DHSS 1986), summarizes the current concept of an appropriate framework of health care.

This form of 'shared' care can have its problems. In Hopkins and Scambler's (1977) community study, for example, for twenty-two visits made by one patient to one hospital, sixteen different signatures were found in the notes, and there was no record of a consultant ever having seen him. Follow-up was generally poor or unrelated to need. Two specific aspects of the medical management of epilepsy are examined here: the use of electroencephalography and anti-convulsant medication. Both were introduced as concepts *within the medical perspective* in the last chapter. The discussion here will focus on the perspectives of people with epilepsy themselves.

a) The role of electroencephalography

Hopkins and Scambler's (1977; 1977a) review of the use made of the EEG amongst their respondents indicated a somewhat ritualistic use of a test which appeared to be of limited value. For fifteen people the records were entirely normal, and a further twenty-four reports contained statements such as 'virtually normal', 'trivial abnormality' or 'probably normal'. If these are included with those reported as entirely normal, then 54 per cent had records that were normal. Two groups were of particular interest: 42 per cent of those having generalized seizures other than *petit mal* monthly or more often had never had an abnormal EEG; and 69 per cent of those with multiple sites of epileptic discharges were having seizures less frequently than monthly.

Few people had a true grasp of the role of electroencephalography in the investigation of epilepsy. Most displayed a partial knowledge; but some were simply confused, a state of affairs for which non-communicative physicians were often held responsible. The following remarks, all from people who had had EEGs, were typical:

It's supposed to make a pattern or something, isn't it?

He said the results were okay and that was it. But I didn't know what they, what all that paperwork involved. They didn't explain nothing.

He said: 'There's something in your brain.' God knows what he meant!

I don't know what they can tell, but they must tell something, mustn't they? They must do.

I don't even know what the heck it's for.

They've never actually told me what the results are, which is a bit frustrating because I like to know these things even if they have to say it in words of one syllable.

I wouldn't know what it was for. It's a marvellous thing, although I nearly fell asleep: I was that comfortable I nearly fell asleep! But whatever it was doing it was just throwing out this . . . it was just throwing out this paper. . . . It was fantastic.

I've no idea what it's for. I'm only a layman. I've no idea, sorry.

Some also reported feeling apprehensive when having EEGs, especially if they were young at the time.

I was very frightened. It's a nerve-racking experience.

I was dead frightened of it. . . . I'd never had that sort of thing done before, you see, and I thought they would electrify me; I kept getting up out of the chair all the time and all that. Next time I went back in the chair and Dad had to come in with me and stay with me.

It may be that the apprehension or fear that some experienced was occasionally due to a conflation of the concepts of EEG and ECT (electroconvulsive therapy). The grounds for this rather alarming suggestion are to be found in the results of a survey of lay opinions about epilepsy (see Scambler 1983). When asked what an EEG is, 39 per cent were aware that it is a medical test somehow related to brain function. Thirty-seven per cent, however, defined it in terms of 'electric shock therapy'. It needs to be remembered, of course, that these individuals, unlike those with epilepsy, had not had the occasion or opportunity to discuss EEGs with a physician.

More striking than either the confusion or apprehension people felt was a tendency to perceive the EEG as a diagnostic test:

They said at the time: 'This will prove whether you've got epilepsy or not.'

We used to more or less think they were blackouts, and then in 1962 I went into this hospital and had some tests in there – the one with the wires – and they said to me: 'These are not blackouts, they're epileptic fits.'

From the accounts proferred, there seemed to be two discernible patterns. First, those who had an EEG *before* they were told they had epilepsy often assumed, or hoped, that a firm diagnosis would follow. Second, those who had an EEG *after* the communication of the diagnosis often hoped, even if they kept it to themselves, that, if normal, it would establish the diagnosis of epilepsy to have been premature and unfounded; in other words, a normal EEG can be numbered among the incentives to disavow a stigmatizing label.

b) Anti-convulsant medication

The importance of patients' perspectives is clearly demonstrated in relation to the 'problem of non-compliance'. It is known that compliance is poor amongst both adults and children with epilepsy – estimates of 40 per cent are common – although it tends to be higher when fewer anti-convulsant drugs are used. Moreover there is some evidence that compliance is not improved by special interventions to inform patients of the value of medication (Pryse-Phillips *et al.* 1982). In one of the few relevant enquiries Schneider and Conrad (1983) have shown that people with epilepsy frequently formulate their own strategies for drug-taking. They found that 'self-regulators' variously altered their prescribed dosages to test out their theories of seizure control; to avoid becoming dependent; to minimize the risk of drug-taking as a stigma cue or as stigmatizing in its own right; to ensure that seizures did not occur on special occasions; or to enhance their sense of control over their conditions.

Three-quarters of those on anti-convulsant medication in Scambler and Hopkins' study said they had always taken their drugs, or, at least, had never deliberately not taken them. In fact, individuals ranged on a continuum from the zealous to the casual drug-taker. Several people described their drug-taking as 'religious': 'I take those tablets religiously.' Another, in the same vein, explained that he took his tablets 'almost like a clock'. At the other end of the continuum were the casual drug-takers:

Sometimes one forgets; sometimes one can't be bothered: whenever possible, you try.

I don't deliberately not take them, but I just don't think of it, you know; I'm too busy.

Sometimes I forget, and sometimes I take it twice; I'm a bit hitty-missy.

A quarter admitted they had at some stage deliberately experimented with or stopped their medication without consulting a physician. One factor which probably facilitated this 'non-compliance' – and which might also have contributed to the conservative prescribing of anti-convulsants and the lack of monitoring of their effects on seizure frequency – was inadequate follow-up. Subsequent audits of care have highlighted this problem (for example, Jones 1980).

An examination of patients' perspectives yielded a number of rationales for experimentation with drug therapy. First, a few people took the initiative in reducing or abandoning therapy as a direct result of negative feelings about taking drugs or because of their effects. Mrs C. just baulked at the idea of swallowing pills: 'I'm a big anti-pill-taker!' Others feared becoming addicted:

Someone told me that if you don't have a turn for a couple of years you don't want to take any more tablets. Well, me not being – I didn't want to become a sort of drug addict, you know, hooked on them, I left them off.

I have myself . . . tried not to get addicted, and I've, without consulting – stupidly, without consulting my doctor – I've tried to cut them down and cut them out myself.

Some people were unhappy with what they defined as side-effects of the drugs. Mr N. was one of several men who felt their sex lives had been diminished since they had been on drugs:

I mean, we have intercourse much like any other couple, and for her it's just the same, but for me it's not, because I know the two differences, as before I took the drugs and afterwards. There's a difference you see.

One in five complained of drowsiness: 'Well, I don't think they're doing anything for me now . . . they're just making me tired and lazy.' Her sister, who was present for part of the interview, added: 'We have to count them every day so she won't try to jump out of taking them!'

Miss G. was another who acknowledged drowsiness and lethargy as side-effects of medication; she had actually had a row with her employer about this on the day she was interviewed:

> My boss intends taking on someone else. I work in a cost office, and I run the cost office at the moment. And he intends to take somebody else for me to teach so *they* can supervise the cost office! And when I asked him why, he said: 'Well, there's always the chance that you're going to have a turn and you won't come in; and when the wages need to be done, if you're not in that day. . . .' So I said to him: 'Well, you've made that point once before, and you were going to give me the sack about six months ago, and I haven't had a day off since.' So he said: 'Yes'. It's sort of hanging in the air at the moment. His explanation, his reason, was that sometimes I seem a little drowsy and he puts it to oneside that I've taken another pill.

She confessed that she was 'not completely with it' if she took a pill midday; for this reason, however, she usually went without one. One-third of those who reported side-effects of drowsiness or impaired concentration had deliberately experimented with their medication, compared with only one in six of those who did not.

A second reason for experimentation was a general disillusionment with therapy. This was often related to the understandable and well-founded conviction that the drugs 'don't cure it, they just control it'. Several found the prospect of taking palliative medication for life, which some physicians unambiguously advocated, depressing and disturbing:

> He just wrote me out a prescription: 'You've got to take these.' Well, I thought that you only had to take them for a few weeks and I said: 'Well, how long do I take them for?' And he said: 'For the rest of your life.' I think that hurt me because I'm not one for taking tablets. . . . It took me a long while before that sank in, because I thought I could take

them one day and leave them off another, until my husband
kept saying: 'You've got to take them. You've got to take
them.'

A policy of drug therapy for life, or for the foreseeable future, was
indicative to many of the unavailability of any effective (curative)
treatment; which was in turn indicative of a profound medical
ignorance about epileptic phenomena.

Medical prognoses tended to be seen as vague and highly
speculative:

He said they might stop when I was 21, or they might stop
when I had my first baby, or they might stop when I reached
'the change'. Well, they didn't stop when I reached 21, so it's
either a case now of my first baby or 'the change', otherwise
I'm going to get them the rest of my life.

They thought that, seven years and you change . . . and when
I was 21 they said they'd change, but they didn't; and after I
had the boy they said they'd go away, but they didn't; and
after I had the girl they said they'd go away, but they still
didn't; and I've still got them.

Miss R. was openly scornful:

They told me that every seven years your body changes. . . .
So I waited seven years after I was 12 [i.e. age at onset] and
when I was 19 I thought: 'Great! Maybe I'll finish with having
my seizures.' Nothing doing. So when you're 19 you say:
'Right, seven years from now I'll be 26: let's see what
happens.' I'm nearly 23, so I've got three years to wait!

When asked if they thought their seizures would cease one day,
38 per cent felt unable to make any prediction; 23 per cent thought
their seizures had already stopped; 15 per cent thought they would
stop one day as a result of medical intervention; 3 per cent thought
they would stop due to some change in their personal or social
circumstances (for example, when they got a job); and 21 per cent
believed they would continue for life. Although most of those
who thought their seizures had ceased had not had one for some
years, a quarter had had some in the year before interview; con-
versely, one in ten of those who thought they would continue for
life had had none for more than six years.

A third reason for changing medication was the pressing desire to shed the status of 'epileptic'. Continuing therapy implied continuing epilepsy, even if there had been no seizures for a number of years. Only if therapy was discontinued would it be possible to determine whether or not the diagnosis of epilepsy was still applicable. The halting of therapy, then, promised possible release from the burden of both recurrent seizures and the diagnostic label. It was such reasoning that prompted remarks like the following:

I really would like to have a go at stopping them altogether, for three or four weeks, just to see what would happen.

Goodness knows, I hope they've stopped. To my way of thinking they've stopped. I would like to stop the tablets and find out!

Unhappily, the assumption shared by many that cessation of seizures and medication would signify a return, first, to a normal health status and, second, to a normal social identity requires some qualification. It is by no means uncommon for an apparent recovery from epilepsy to turn into a remission. And stigmatizing labels have a habit of outliving the attributes, traits, or conditions they initially denote. As Freidson puts it:

unlike other imputed qualities, stigma is by definition ineradicable and irreversible: it is so closely connected with identity that even after the cause of the imputation of stigma has been removed and the social reaction has been ostensibly redirected, identity is formed by the fact of *having* been in a stigmatized role: the cured mental patient is not just another person, but an ex-mental patient; the rehabilitated criminal gone straight is an ex-convict. One's identity is permanently spoiled.

(Freidson 1970: 236)

A note on patients' perspectives

One of the central themes of this chapter has been that it is short-sighted to analyse physician–patient relationships or exchanges on the assumption that physicians are active and patients passive. The great majority of patients must be classed as active: as the discussions of responses to the diagnosis of epilepsy, of attempts to make sense of epilepsy, and of the role of electroencephalography and of anti-convulsant medication have suggested, they develop their own ideas and attitudes concerning epilepsy and its medical management which are not always in accordance with those propagated by their physicians.

The single most important source of the often latent conflict between the perspectives of physicians and patients is probably the perception of epilepsy as a stigmatizing condition. In Scambler and Hopkins' work, for example, it was this at times overriding perception which variously prompted patients to reject the diagnosis of epilepsy, or at least to negotiate for a less virulent alternative; to misinterpret or reinterpret normal EEGs as evidence of premature or mistaken diagnosis; and to defy medical advice about drug-taking in order to hasten the transition from 'epileptic' to 'normal' status.

This sense of stigma also led many patients to take umbrage at what they interpreted as physicians' preoccupation with the diagnosis and treatment of disease. Miss G. was provoked to say:

> I don't think doctors understand how you feel. I think they understand it medically to a certain extent, but I don't think they understand your problem mentally in trying to cope with the fact that you have them [i.e. seizures], and to cope with, sort of, life.

This charge that physicians lacked the inclination, skill or time to show empathy – and hence volunteered little or no information or counsel on the psycho-social sequelae of epilepsy – was most often directed at hospital specialists. Mr W. described them as essentially 'academic'. And Mrs M.'s comment was typical:

> I think all they're interested in is finding the drug that will curtail it, as much as it can, with as few side-effects as possible. . . . I never felt there was any help as regards coping with the fits themselves or the side-effects *they* had. They didn't ask you how you managed your life around them.

West (1985) has referred to a 'conspiracy of silence' in which physicians appear uninterested, insecure, hurried, and unable to discuss patients' problems. Elsewhere he suggests that what they lack is a coherent 'stigma ideology' in relation to epilepsy: in particular, they have no clear 'set of prescriptions, or "practice theories", to enable the stigmatized themselves to manage their situation as effectively as possible' (West 1979: 647). One result of this, he believes, is that 'the physician is in danger of legitimating the stigma of epilepsy, not by talking about it, but by *not* talking about it' (1979: 652).

It would be misleading to imply, however, that people with epilepsy are altogether unsympathetic to the medical management of their conditions. In fact, in Scambler and Hopkins' study, there was often a deep tension within patients' perspectives on medical involvement. On the one hand, their desire and determination to avoid the stigmatizing status of 'epileptic' led them to contest or equivocate over medical pronouncements and advice and to baulk at the narrow, biomedical preoccupation with disease. On the other hand they acknowledged, almost without exception, that the physicians they had consulted were – if occasionally flawed and certainly not omniscient – experts, unlike themselves, and that they therefore 'knew best'. Mr P. was by no means uncritical of the care he had received, and yet concluded with: 'These things are best left to the professionals.' Typically, people seemed to vacillate between these two contradictory positions in the light of their immediate circumstances.

Chapter three

Lay concepts of epilepsy and stigma

It is already apparent that many people with epilepsy regard their condition as highly stigmatizing, and that this perception can shape their careers as patients. In fact individuals with epilepsy and physicians typically coincide in their assessments of the public image of epilepsy and 'epileptics' as deeply negative. It would perhaps not be surprising if these assessments were accurate. Temkin (1945) has shown that throughout history, inside as well as outside 'medicine', epilepsy has been subject to demonological interpretation and sufferers to ritualistic and institutional abuse. In contemporary Third World cultures, epileptic phenomena continue to be defined in supernatural terms. A recent community study in Nigeria, for example, found that, after heredity, 'witchcraft' was the cause most commonly attributed to epilepsy amongst the lay populace (Awaritefe *et al.* 1985). Danesi (1984) has revealed that most Nigerians with epilepsy experience it as highly stigmatizing and something to be hidden from others.

Contemporary lay thinking about epilepsy

What, then, is the public image of epilepsy in the modern industrial or post-industrial cultures of Europe and the US? It is clearly important to know whether or not the somewhat pessimistic judgements about lay thinking by people with epilepsy and their physicians are justified. Most patients and physicians hold what has been called the 'orthodox viewpoint' on lay thinking (Scambler and Hopkins 1986). This viewpoint is reflected in the following passage from the 'Reid Report' of 1969:

Through ignorance and prejudice about the nature of the

disease, there is a reluctance to give them a home, a job, or to accept them as relations by marriage or as fit to become natural or adoptive parents.

(CHSC 1969: 16)

More analytically, the orthodox viewpoint may be said to consist of four theses, namely, that the public is ignorant about what epilepsy is; intolerant in its attitudes towards sufferers; prone to discriminatory practices against them; and responsible for most of the problems associated with an epileptic identity. Each will be considered in turn.

Three erroneous beliefs are often said to epitomize public ignorance. The first is the definition of epilepsy solely in terms of *grand mal* seizures; the second is the classification of epilepsy as a type of mental disorder; and the third is the association of epilepsy with the possession of numerous and varied anti-social personality traits.

A community survey conducted amongst adults in Windsor and utilizing semi-structured interviews found that 54 per cent of respondents defined epilepsy exclusively in terms of its most dramatic manifestation, the *grand mal* seizure, a proportion somewhat lower than many would have predicted (Scambler 1983). In a more recent street survey of people aged 16–45 in London using highly structured interviews, when asked to describe an 'epileptic attack', 67 per cent gave descriptions consistent with a *grand mal* seizure. However, when asked subsequently if there was more than one type of epileptic seizure, 71 per cent answered in the affirmative (Jordan *et al.* 1986). It may well be the case that people's *initial* response to epilepsy is in terms of the *grand mal* seizure, despite the fact that many of them are aware that there are alternative types of seizure. Predictably perhaps, there is some indirect evidence that the association in people's minds between the terms 'fit' and 'grand mal' is stronger than that between 'epilepsy/epileptic attack' and 'grand mal' (Harrison and West 1977).

The belief that epilepsy is a form of mental disorder has been widely researched throughout Europe and the US. The Windsor study found 16 per cent categorizing epilepsy as a mental disorder. Twenty-five per cent in the London street survey saw epilepsy as a mental as opposed to a physical disorder, although some clearly did so only because the brain was the part of the body affected. In Harrison and West's street survey in Bristol and Oxford, relying on semi-structured interviews, 11 per cent apparently regarded people with epilepsy as 'mental types' (i.e. disturbed, 'mental' or having a psychiatric problem).

A number of large-scale surveys using questionnaires rather than interviews have also been conducted and bear on this issue. Table 3.1 summarizes the relevant data from a sequence of studies carried out in the US at five-yearly intervals since 1949, and from comparable studies in West Germany, Britain and Italy. In each of these studies the question was posed: 'Do you think epilepsy is a form of insanity, or not?' Responses in the US suggest a gradual increase in lay awareness since the Second World War: 13 per cent regarded epilepsy as a form of insanity in 1949, compared with only 3 per cent thirty years later. The equivalent figures for West Germany – 23 per cent in 1967 falling to 21 per cent in 1978 – seem particularly high. Various reasons have been proferred for this. For example, Janz (1969) suggested of the 1967 figure that it may owe something to the Nazi eugenic laws which classified epilepsy and mental disorder in the same category, and also to the fact that until quite recently psychiatry and neurology were considered one academic discipline in Germany.

Table 3.1 Comparison of international survey responses to the question: 'Do you think epilepsy is a form of insanity, or not?'

Year	Yes (%)	No (%)	Don't know/not familiar with epilepsy (%)
US studies			
1949	13	59	28
1954	7	68	25
1959	4	74	22
1964	4	79	17
1969	4	81	15
1974	2	86	12
1979	3	92	5
West German studies			
1967	23	50	27
1978	21	68	11
British study			
1969	6	76	18
Italian study			
1983	5	58	37

Source: Adapted from Canger and Cornaggia 1985

The notion that epilepsy is linked in the lay imagination with a series of negative personality characteristics is ironical in that, as Bagley argues, 'physicians themselves have been guilty of prejudice against epilepsy. Many authors of papers have attributed negative and anti-social traits to the epileptic when the canons of scientific knowledge ought to have restrained them from doing so' (1971: 108). Even after Tizard (1962) finally debunked the myth of the 'epileptic personality', the term continued and continues to be utilized in medical texts and circles (see Chapter 4).

In the Windsor study of lay opinion, 18 per cent felt people with epilepsy tend to have undesirable personality traits; those mentioned being excitability, aggressiveness and weakness. The equivalent figure in the London street survey was 16 per cent. Interestingly, the street survey in Bristol and Oxford produced a very different finding. Harrison and West offer a 'conservative' estimate that as many as 52 per cent 'attributed one or more negative traits to epileptics in general' (West 1979: 263). The personality 'types' identified by at least one in ten were: violent/aggressive (21 per cent), nervy (17 per cent), highly-strung/unstable (12 per cent), mental (11 per cent) and withdrawn/timid (10 per cent). But they add: 'There is not, however, substantial agreement between them as to what sort of person the typical sufferer is. . . . There is therefore no *one* public stereotype but a series of overlapping "negative" images about epileptic identity' (West 1979: 263). There is no ready explanation for the difference between this result and those of the Windsor and London surveys.

A summary of the research literature on these three putative lay beliefs about epilepsy might run as follows. Although ignorance and error persist, most studies suggest they are less prevalent than advocates of the orthodox viewpoint have claimed, and are diminishing. Moreover there is clearly no single, pervasive or cultural stereotype of 'the epileptic'. In the Windsor study, for example, only one of the eighty-five respondents held all three erroneous beliefs, and only a further six some combination of two of them.

The Windsor, London, and Bristol/Oxford surveys all found little evidence of antagonistic attitudes towards people with epilepsy amongst the lay population. Indeed, statements of sympathy and tolerance were commonplace. The questionnaire-based studies conducted in the US, West Germany, Britain and Italy included the following question: 'Would you object to having any of your children in school or at play associate with persons who sometimes had seizures (fits)?' The replies are presented in Table 3.2. It is noticeable that the studies in the US indicate enhanced tolerance over time, with the percentages responding with a 'yes' falling from 24 per cent in 1949 to 6 per cent in 1979. Once again the equivalent figures in West Germany seem high, falling from 31 per cent in 1967 to 21 per cent in 1978.

Table 3.2 Comparison of international survey responses to the question: 'Would you object to having any of your children in school or at play associate with persons who sometimes had seizures (fits)?'

Year	Yes %	No %	Don't know/not familiar with epilepsy %
US studies			
1949	24	57	19
1954	17	68	15
1959	18	67	15
1964	13	77	10
1969	9	81	10
1974	5	84	11
1979	6	89	5
West German studies			
1967	31	42	27
1978	21	68	11
British study			
1969	15	68	17
Italian study			
1983	8	58	34

Source: Adapted from Canger and Cornaggia 1985

The same studies also incorporated a question on employment: 'Do you think epileptics should be employed in jobs like other people?' As Table 3.3 shows, the proportions replying negatively have decreased in the US from 35 per cent in 1949 to 9 per cent in 1979.

The bulk of the published research on lay opinions on epilepsy and its sufferers would seem to support this picture of increased tolerance, as well as increased knowledge, since the war. There are, however, three important qualifications to be made. First, many of the relevant studies have relied either on very highly structured interviews or on questionnaires, and these share certain disadvantages as instruments of research. For example, not all questions can be reasonably answered within the framework of a finite number of choices. Consider the question: 'Do you think

Table 3.3 Comparison of international survey responses to the question: 'Do you think epileptics should be employed in jobs like other people?'

Year	Yes %	No %	Don't know/not familiar with epilepsy %
US studies			
1949	45	35	20
1954	60	22	18
1959	75	11	14
1964	82	9	9
1969	76	12	12
1974	81	8	11
1979	79	9	12
West German studies			
1967	45	26	29
1978	70	18	12
British study			
1969	57	23	20
Italian study			
1983	51	11	38

Source: Adapted from Canger and Cornaggia 1985

epileptics should be employed in jobs like other people?' Although the principal author of the 1949–1979 American studies, Caveness, has acknowledged a tendency among respondents to want to *qualify* their answers (for example, 'if treated for the disease', 'if capable', 'if some plan is provided to prevent injury'), his reports only allow for an unqualified 'yes', 'no', or 'don't know' (Caveness *et al*, 1969). It is unclear how such forced replies are to be interpreted.

Two related findings from the London street survey are pertinent here. It also incorporated this same employment question, and 6 per cent felt that people with epilepsy should not be employed in jobs like others, compared with the latest American figure of 9 per cent. However, when a Lickert scale was used to measure participants' agreement or disagreement with the statement 'Some jobs are unsuitable for people with epilepsy', 29 per cent 'strongly agreed', 62 per cent 'agreed', and 9 per cent 'didn't know'; not a single person disagreed with the statement. It is clear in this instance, therefore, that lay persons' almost unanimous acceptance of people with epilepsy's right to work was strictly conditional on the nature of the work.

Second, a few studies have produced results which appear to contradict the trend to greater enlightenment and toleration. For example, Bagley (1972), using a social distance scale, found there is still considerable public antagonism towards people with epilepsy in Britain. One of his findings was that people with epilepsy are more often rejected than those with either cerebral palsy or mental illness. He adds, with acknowledged irony, that if more people saw epilepsy as a form of insanity this might make sufferers more rather than less acceptable. Interestingly, a similar study carried out in the US a decade later, also using a social distance scale, found that people with epilepsy are less often rejected than those with cerebral palsy or mental illness (Albrecht *et al.* 1982). It is unclear how apparently opposing results like these are to be interpreted. Are they explicable in terms of the time gap between the two studies, or in terms of the different cultures in which the studies were conducted?

The third qualification is in many ways the most significant. It has long been known that beliefs and attitudes are poor predictors of behaviour. It was imprudent of the authors of the 'Reid Report', therefore, to infer a high rate of lay discrimination against people with epilepsy solely on the basis of a prior – and, as it turns out, largely unwarranted – commitment to the theses of extensive public ignorance and verbally expressed intolerance. Similarly, it would be unwise to infer that discrimination is diminishing or dying out solely on the basis of evidence obtained from highly structured surveys indicating a gradual enhancement of lay knowledge and sympathy since the Second World War.

This leads on to a necessarily brief consideration of the third and fourth component theses of the orthodox viewpoint, namely, that members of the public are prone to discriminate against people with epilepsy, and that this is the principal cause of the problems accompanying an epileptic status. There is in fact no worthwhile empirical evidence, in either Europe or the US, for or against these theses. Indeed, there is an urgent need for studies of discriminatory practices and their effects which deploy convincing measures of discrimination and are independent of putative victims' accounts. These would almost certainly incorporate comparison groups of people without epilepsy. While it is undoubtedly true, then, that most physicians and others concerned with the health and well-being of people with epilepsy have a batch of 'horror stories' to relate, these cannot count as evidence either that public discrimination is rampant or that it is the cause of widespread disruption or despondency. There is simply no way of estimating how representative these stories are.

A reasonable summary of research relating to the orthodox viewpoint, a viewpoint held by many physicians as well as people with epilepsy, might be couched in the following terms. There is some evidence that lay knowledge of epilepsy is increasing and attitudes towards sufferers mellowing. It does not follow, however, that lay discrimination based on stigma is a thing of the past. In fact there is as yet no reliable evidence indicating either the prevalence of such discrimination against people with epilepsy or its impact on their biographies. If the first two theses of the orthodox viewpoint are at best dubious, the second pair are mere conjecture.

Discrimination based on stigma

Although nothing may be known about rates of discriminatory practices based on stigma, there is no doubt either that such practices still occur or that their effects on individuals can be devastating. For this reason, and because of physicians' and sufferers' continuing commitment to the orthodox viewpoint, it is worth asking why people with epilepsy may meet with avoidance and rejection. The question is the one posed by Scott in relation to blind people: 'why individuals should be labelled deviant and excluded from full participation in the community when there is nothing in their behaviour to warrant this kind of treatment?' (1972: 13). The essence of Scott's answer is that the blind and others like them constitute a threat to the social order (Scambler 1984). But just how might people with epilepsy threaten the social order? Three views will be considered here.

The first, proposed by Bagley, maintains that there exists 'an innate prejudice against epilepsy' which is rooted in a fear that the sufferer is always liable to sudden, unpredictable and dramatic losses of motor control, to 'going berserk' (something which normal people fear in themselves). The individual with epilepsy differs from someone with, say, cerebral palsy in that the latter's loss of motor control is constant (and therefore predictable) and mild. Bagley adds:

> The prejudiced observer of epilepsy may ask himself the implicit question: 'If he can maintain control of himself for days, weeks, or months, why can't he control himself now?' The victim of cerebral palsy cannot be blamed in this way, for he has never 'gained' control of himself, and so he cannot lose it. He is not 'morally' responsible.
>
> (1971: 113)

Much of this, as Bagley confesses, has never been empirically examined; but he does elsewhere claim a limited measure of support from his finding that people with epilepsy are 'much more often rejected' than are those with cerebral palsy (Bagley 1972). Against this of course may be cited the contrary finding of Albrecht and colleagues mentioned earlier.

The second account, by Taylor, was constructed in response to the question: 'Why is epilepsy socially unacceptable?' Taylor argues, in the manner of Scott, that

> the social structure survives through its experience of the value of control, order and reason. Circumstances which threaten loss of control provoke a strong social reaction, be they in crowd behaviour or in the activities of a deviant group, or in alcohol excess, or drug intoxication.
>
> (Taylor 1969: 107)

Two circumstances, Taylor contends, are especially threatening to control over the environment: madness and death. He continues:

> If we were without any medical knowledge and observed the phenomenon of epilepsy, we would observe in an epileptic fit a brief excursion through madness into death. Normally, there are complex social mechanisms for dealing with these eventualities, grief, mourning, rejection, and so on. The psychological difficulty in accepting epilepsy is that the fit having severed human relationships in this way is followed by recovery; that it does this recurrently involves the constant reformation of the status quo ante. Every fit reinforces the view of witnesses that the epileptic cannot be relied upon to participate fully in society, since he is liable, at any time, to

go out of control. Therefore, unless he can be cured, he must be set apart; he must be reformed, or else rejected.

(1969: 107)

Not surprisingly perhaps, Taylor offers no empirical backing for these views.

The third view, put forward by Scambler (1983; 1984), suggests that the person with epilepsy threatens the social order in two main ways. First, he or she fails to conform to cultural norms pertaining to what Goffman calls 'identity or being'. Goffman writes:

Failure or success at maintaining such norms has a very direct effect on the psychological integrity of the individual. At the same time, mere desire to abide by the norm – mere good will – is not enough, for in many cases the individual has no immediate control over his level of sustaining the norm. It is a question of the individual's condition, not his will; it is a question of conformance, not compliance.

(1968: 152–3)

Of epilepsy itself, Goffman notes in passing that since Hippocrates' time 'those who discover they have this disorder have been assured a firmly stigmatized self by the definitional workings of society. This work still goes on even though insignificant physical impairment may be involved' (1968: 150). It could be said that the person with epilepsy in contemporary societies like Britain and the US possesses an *ontological deficit*. It is not that such a person stands condemned for some kind of wrongdoing – there is no *moral* culpability – but rather that he or she is an imperfect being. Freidson writes:

What is analytically peculiar about the assignment of stigma is the fact that while a stigmatized person need not be held responsible for what is imputed to him, nonetheless, somewhat like those to whom responsibility is imputed, he is denied the ordinary privileges of social life.

(1970: 235)

Scott writes similarly of the lot of the blind: 'it became apparent to me that there were many blind people who were regarded a social deviants, simply because they could not see; their behaviour had nothing at all to do with it' (1972: 13). According to this view, then, and against Bagley's, people with epilepsy are rarely 'blamed' or held to be either morally or causally responsible for their seizures (although it may feel like it at times).

Second, people with epilepsy threaten the social order by causing what Albrecht and colleagues refer to as *ambiguity in social interaction*. In their study of the attitudes of normal people this was 'the most frequent reason given for distancing from the stigmatized' (1982: 1324). One may hypothesize that there are three principal and closely related dimensions to the disruption or ambiguity in social interaction provoked by the individual with epilepsy. The first concerns the instability or *unpredictability* inherent in epilepsy. Bagley writes, for example, of the lay person's fear of 'apparently uncontrollable impulses suddenly manifesting themselves' (1972: 38). The second is the *drama* of losses of control when they do occur, particularly with *grand mal* (which may or may not be aptly described by Taylor as 'a brief excursion through madness into death'). It might be objected here that there are many other types of epileptic seizure, and that more members of the public are aware of this than many commentators have assumed. Nevertheless, nine out of every ten participants in Hopkins and Scambler's (1977) community study had had a generalized seizure other than *petit mal* at some time in their lives.

The third dimension is a *fear of coping*, or, more precisely, of having to assume responsibility for someone having a seizure. This is perhaps the least striking of the three dimensions to ambiguity in social interaction, but may well be the most significant. There are two main aspects to fear of coping. The first is 'ignorance' about what exactly is happening and about what ought to be done. Albrecht and colleagues write of their study:

> Various respondents stated: 'We are usually afraid of those things which we don't understand and things that are new or foreign to us'; 'The person doesn't know how to cope and feels uncomfortable with the disabled'; and 'they don't know what, if anything, they should do to help'. Rejection of the stigmatized persons and their subsequent rebuff by normal adults was believed to result from ignorance about the disabled person's condition and not knowing how to interact or when to help.
>
> (1982: 1324)

The second is a feeling of 'impotence', akin in many ways to the sense of helplessness experienced by members of sufferers' own families on witnessing onset (see Chapter 5). Seizures cannot be arrested, and help which consists in doing nothing, or very little, does not seem much like help at all, especially if the seizure is dramatic or bizarre.

Of course while some practise discrimination against people with epilepsy on grounds of stigma, others do not. It would be foolhardy to attempt an a priori identification of types of people likely to discriminate here, but two areas might repay examination. The first centres on 'personality'. It seems reasonable to suppose that those who discriminate – specifically in relation to epilepsy, and generally in relation to all forms of 'ascribed deviance' – are themselves vulnerable, that the disdain and hostility they display in their behaviour towards people with epilepsy are indicative of a deficiency in their own capacity to cope with uncertainty and contingency. And the second area involves what Goffman calls 'courtesy stigma', one aspect of the 'disabling of the normal' (Hilbourne 1973). Goffman writes: 'the tendency for a stigma to spread from the stigmatized individual to his close connexions provides a reason why such relations tend either to be avoided or to be terminated, where existing' (1968: 43). It may be the case that some discriminate in order to preclude the possibility that the 'stigma of epilepsy' will spread to them.

Legitimate discrimination

Discrimination based on stigma is not of course the sole prerogative of the individual. Institutions, including the law, can and have exercised this same function. Until 1965, for example, prohibition against people with epilepsy marrying was still operational in some American states. Indeed, it was not until 1980 that Missouri finally removed its law forbidding such marriages. As recently as 1978 Arkansas and Missouri permitted the annulment of an adoption if the child developed epilepsy within five years (see Dell 1986). It is necessary, however, to distinguish further between individual and institutional discrimination based on stigma and what might be called 'legitimate' discrimination. There are contexts in which all parties – people with epilepsy, physicians, the public and its representatives – accept the case for limited discrimination against those with epilepsy. The most obvious example is driving.

The accident rate amongst licensed drivers with epilepsy is 1.3 to 2.0 times that amongst age-matched controls without epilepsy. But the regulations in force vary enormously both between and within different countries. The current UK regulations came into effect in 1982 as a result of *The Motor Vehicles (Driving Licences) (Amendment) (No. 3) Regulations:*

> Epilepsy is prescribed for the purposes of section 87 (3) (b) of the Act of 1972 and an applicant for a licence suffering from epilepsy shall satisfy the conditions that – (a) he shall have been free from any epileptic attack during the period of two years immediately preceding the date when the licence is to come into effect; or (b) in the case of an applicant who has had such attacks whilst asleep during that period, he shall have had such attacks only whilst asleep during a period of at least three years immediately preceding the date when the licence is to have effect; and (c) the driving of a vehicle by him in pursuance of the licence is not likely to be a source of danger to the public.

People presenting after a single seizure will lose their licence for one year, unless there is a predictable continuing liability to seizures, in which event they will not regain it until they have been free from seizures for two years. This requirement is not specified in the Regulations, but, under (c) above, is applied at the discretion of the Secretary of State for the Environment on advice from the Driving and Vehicles Licencing Centre. It is to the latter body that patients in the UK who have had either a single seizure or developed epilepsy are obliged to report. Nobody can hold a licence entitling them to drive heavy goods vehicles or public service vehicles such as buses if they had any epileptic event of any type, isolated or multiple, after the age of five (Hopkins and Harvey 1987).

Many people, of course, put a high premium on the ability to drive, and sometimes their jobs depend on it. Moreover, as Hopkins and Scambler found (Scambler 1983), not being able to drive can be stigmatizing in its own right:

> Unless you are actually in the position where you suffer from it, you can't . . . it's very difficult to understand the limitations that are placed on your life. As I say, I can't drive.

It doesn't sound much, but a 30-year-old publican who can't drive is enough of an enigma to be remarked upon constantly.

Nor did this man feel able to explain why he had no licence:

People say: 'Well, why don't you drive?' And you have to start inventing excuses. You can't afford – you see, there's still a certain amount of social stigma, a large amount of social stigma on epilepsy; and you can't afford to turn round and say to the public at large: 'I don't drive because I'm an epileptic', because, as far as they're concerned, an epileptic is a lunatic.

In one community study, two-thirds of those interviewed were ineligible to drive. Of the sixty-two individuals ineligible to drive, eighteen acknowledged that they had been diagnosed as suffering from epilepsy and said they had been advised by their physician not to drive: three were in fact driving. A further five insisted that the diagnosis of epilepsy had not been made but admitted they had been advised not to drive: two were driving. Four said they had been told by a physician that they could drive and four felt they had received his or her implicit consent: seven were driving. The remaining 31 of those ineligible to drive, most of whom had never driven and all of whom were not driving when interviewed, said they had received ambivalent or no advice about driving. In sum, one in five of those ineligible to drive were driving (Hopkins and Scambler 1977; Scambler 1983).

Extrapolating from these figures, only just over a third of those ineligible to drive said they recollected receiving unambiguous medical advice not to drive. Two points need to be borne in mind. First, in some instances physicians may have thought such advice redundant. And second, recall of medical advice generally is known to be poor (and maybe especially poor when the advice is unwelcome). It seems likely, however, that a number of physicians were less than clear in their interpretation and exposition of the regulations governing epilepsy and driving (see Harvey and Hopkins 1983). Miss F., who did not drive after onset, recounted her experiences with some bitterness:

I was cross with my doctor . . . I was told that: 'I think perhaps you oughtn't to drive.' It seemed – as I'd actually been driving when I had this blackout – sensible, so I didn't drive; and my doctor said: 'Perhaps you'd better not drive for a year.' I

said: 'Alright, I won't drive for a year', and didn't re-insure
the car, and put it away. And at the end of the year I went
to see him and said: 'Look, I've been alright for a year: no
episodes, no blackouts, no nothing. Can I drive?' 'Oh', he
said, 'I will refer back to the specialist, I'll ask him. I'll discuss
it with him.' And he evidently did, because then he wrote
and said that Dr X (i.e. the specialist) agrees that you shouldn't
drive, that you should give it another year.' So: 'Alright, I'll
give it another year.' And again I went to him, and I said:
'Look, I've done two years now. Can I drive?'

She was then told by her general practitioner that she must write
to 'the licensing people' and explain her position. 'Like a fool',
she did. They immediately asked for her licence, informing her
that there was a minimum wait of three years (amended to two
years in 1982). 'That did irk me. At first it was a voluntary one
year, then a voluntary two years, and now it's a highly involuntary
three years!'

When the law was explained to them during the course of the
interviews, most of those who had driven illegally accepted that
the law was justified: 'I think the law is right. I think I'm chancing
my arm a bit.' 'Well, in a sense it is right, because you're endangering the public – just like me, I'm endangering the public. . . .
So I suppose they're right stopping you from driving.' There
seemed little doubt, however, that *all* would continue driving. As
one man put it: 'I mean, a car is like your right arm, isn't it?'

Chapter four

Strategies for coping and their effects

Not all authors agree that people with epilepsy's sense of stigma is pervasive and debilitating. Ryan *et al.* (1980) have claimed that many sufferers in the US do not feel this way. For example, as many as four out of five of those who completed postal question-naires felt they had been treated fairly by employers. About 70 per cent felt they had been neither unduly restricted nor treated differently as a result of their seizures. It may be significant, however, that the index of 'perceived stigma' developed by Ryan and her associates contained several items on whether or not respondents had actually *experienced* discrimination based on stigma. In her report of her general study of disability in Britain, Blaxter included this comment:

> Epilepsy came into a special category. In fact, none of the sample's epileptics gave any evidence at all that they had experienced any social stigma, but each one expressed surprise and gratitude at this and told generalized stories about the problems which epileptics 'usually' faced.
>
> (1976: 198)

This suggests that it may be useful to distinguish between expect-ing or fearing discrimination and actually experiencing it. Just such a distinction arose out of the work of Scambler and Hopkins (1986).

Felt and enacted stigma

Stebbins (1970) has suggested that the way individuals interpret events and happenings – past, present and future – associated with a particular identity often evolves into a 'special view of the world'. Whenever this identity becames salient to them, their 'special view of the world' predisposes them to a patterned response. Scambler and Hopkins argue that the people with epilepsy in their study typically possessed a 'special view of the world' in this sense. Moreover, essentially the same perceptions characterized people's 'special view of the world' at the time of interview as had characterized their initial responses to the communication of the diagnosis. Most significantly, they persisted in their definition of epilepsy as stigmatizing. Members of the public still stood convicted of ignorance, error, hostility, and discrimination based on stigma. Eighty-four per cent of those interviewed went out of their way to emphasize lay ignorance about epilepsy, and exactly the same proportion made explicit and unsolicited statements about the social and cultural unacceptability of 'being epileptic'. Miss R., a 22-year-old secretary, spoke for this majority:

> People are ignorant of epilepsy. I don't mean 'ignorant' rudely: I mean they're ignorant of the word epilepsy. The word epilepsy is like cancer, the word cancer; they hate the word and they don't understand what's behind it. . . . If someone mentions the word epilepsy – and once or twice I've caught someone saying: 'Oh, you know that person who suffers from, you know, that thing, where they have those convulsions' – I have to defend myself saying: 'Well, I have a friend. . . .' I defend myself through an invisible friend, because I can't say to them: 'Well, I have that', without knowing damn well that I'd get sacked, and that they'd give me a very, very smug excuse for it.

These deeply felt remarks could almost be read as an affirmation of the orthodox viewpoint assessed and found wanting in the last chapter.

It will be helpful at this stage to introduce a distinction between *enacted* and *felt* stigma (Scambler 1984; Scambler and Hopkins 1986). Enacted stigma refers to episodes of discrimination against people with epilepsy solely on the grounds of their social and cultural unacceptability. This specifically excludes instances of discrimination widely perceived as reasonable, and defined in the previous chapter as 'legitimate' (for example, bans on driving trains or operating heavy industrial machinery). Felt stigma has two referents. The first is the shame associated with having epilepsy. Scambler and Hopkins suggest that this derives less from any sense of moral culpability than from an often unarticulated feeling that epilepsy is evidence of imperfection, of a spoiled identity or being (Goffman 1968). They found that epilepsy was typically seen as an ontological deficit rather than a moral one. The second and most significant referent is, simply, the fear of encountering enacted stigma.

Drawing on this distinction, a model which has greater explanatory potential than the orthodox viewpoint has been constructed (Scambler and Hopkins 1986). This will be termed the *hidden distress* model. It can be epitomized in three propositions:

(a) When a physician communicates the diagnosis of epilepsy to them people quickly learn to regard the status of 'epileptic' as a social liability. In general terms this is because they come to define epilepsy as stigmatizing; more specifically, it has its origin in a characteristic 'special view of the world' in which a fear of enacted stigma predominates.

(b) This 'special view of the world' predisposes people, above all else, to hide their condition and its medical diagnosis from others, to attempt to pass as 'normal'. The fear of enacted stigma promotes a policy of non-disclosure, a policy which remains viable for as long as people are 'discreditable' rather than 'discredited' (Goffman 1968).

(c) This policy of strict concealment reduces the opportunities for, and hence rate of, enacted stigma, most notably in the context of personal relationships and work. One important consequence of this is that felt stigma, and especially the fear of enacted stigma, is more disruptive of the lives of people with epilepsy than enacted stigma.

As explained in the last chapter, one outstanding question remains unanswered, namely, to what extent is felt stigma justified? The degree of risk of enacted stigma is unknown.

It may be helpful to illustrate the hidden distress model with an extended case study (Scambler and Hopkins 1986: 39–42). Ralph S. was a married man aged 29 when interviewed. He experienced his first *petit mal* seizure at the age of 4. His parents took him to their general practitioner and he was referred for neurological assessment. The diagnosis of epilepsy was made and communicated to Ralph's parents, although he knew nothing of it himself until after his first *grand mal* seizure at the age of 18. In the course of the investigation of his *petit mal* seizures his mother discovered that her husband had suffered from epilepsy prior to their marriage. It was she who determined that Ralph's epilepsy should remain a secret: shared only with her sister. Ralph's brother, two years younger than him, did not learn of the diagnosis until Ralph did. Ralph recalled: 'My mother would never allow the word epilepsy to be used in any way, shape or form by anyone, even family, doctors, teachers, whatever!' His seizures were known in the immediate family as 'dreams'. Reflecting on his mother's behaviour, Ralph said: 'Because of the social stigma that is still attached to the disease, I think I would act in just the same manner.'

He left school at the age of 15 and soon after began an apprenticeship in the printing industry. This involved regular attendance at a printing college, and it was here that he had his first *grand mal* seizure at the age of 18. An ambulance was called and he was taken to hospital where, 'having suspected it for a while', he asked the specialist 'straight out' if he had epilepsy: 'I was half afraid to have it confirmed.' The diagnosis was confirmed. Encouraged by his mother, who reiterated the need for absolute secrecy, his sense of felt stigma became acute. He was upset also when he was told he would not be able to drive for a number of years. Nor could he explain to his various friends *why* he would be unable to obtain a licence. Although several friends had known about his 'dreams' and come to accept them, only one or two close, trusted friends were eventually informed of the diagnosis. Ralph felt he was very fortunate in that no friends ever witnessed one of his *grand mal* seizures, which he clearly thought would have given his epilepsy away. His *petit mal* seizures gradually reduced in frequency, from one or more a day in early childhood to less than one a year at the time of interview.

Ralph had his first *grand mal* seizure at college on a Thursday and returned to work the following Monday, the only time he has ever been absent from work because of his epilepsy. He said nothing about the diagnosis of epilepsy and, 'luckily', had no additional seizures at work. He completed his apprenticeship and took employment briefly as a printer with two firms. He had no seizures at work during this period and again made no disclosures. By the age of 23, however, he had become frustrated with printing and determined to train as a publican. He travelled the country as a trainee manager for a year or more, again experiencing no seizures at work and making no disclosures. He had taken over managership of his second public house a few months before taking part in the study.

While Ralph was a trainee manager he met his future wife, herself a trainee on the same scheme. He had had a number of girlfriends before, but had never had a seizure in their presence and had always successfully passed as 'normal'. When the relationship deepened and marriage became a possibility, he felt obliged to disclose fully. Despite his apprehension, induced by felt stigma, she seemed to receive the news well and showed no signs of wanting to break the relationship off. Nor was there any negative reaction when Ralph told her parents of his epilepsy and their plans to marry. His wife explained that she actually witnessed one of Ralph's *grand mal* seizures after his disclosure but before they married. They were playing cards in his parents' home at the time, while his parents watched television in an adjacent room. She said she was 'frightened' because she had never seen one before and 'had no idea what to do'; she called out to his parents. Ralph's mother later told her that she had thought this would put an end to their plans to marry: 'She was quite surprised to see me back the next day!' A few months later they married.

Ralph felt his epilepsy had not intruded much on married life. In the early days they had had protracted discussions about his seizures and their implications, but both thought the subject just about 'exhausted' and said they only dwelt on it now when he actually had a seizure. When Ralph's wife became pregnant, however, they worried that a child might inherit the disorder and sought medical counsel; they were told they could only 'wait and see'. At the time of interview their son was 19 months old and, 'touch wood', in perfect health. It was Ralph's firm intention that he would never learn that this father had (had) epilepsy. Although he said he detested having to 'lead a life of secrecy', he still judged it to be necessary, given the public image of the person with epilepsy: 'It's a person who throws fits and goes mad.'

If a state of equilibrium in the family was proving fairly easy to maintain, at least while Ralph's son was so small, the maintenance of equilibrium at work was a much more precarious business. He felt he tended to have seizures when under pressure, and events and circumstances which led him to feel tense often functioned as 'situational stimuli' which prompted him to dwell on his condition and retreat into the 'special view of the world' rooted in felt stigma. He was especially anxious about the possibility of a *grand mal* seizure in a crowded bar. Apart from being 'shameful' in its own right, this would almost certainly expose him as 'an epileptic' to his clients, in which instance: 'I would personally feel that my authority had been undermined.' Moreover his employers might get to hear of it and then his job would be at risk: 'Whoever heard of a publican with epilepsy?' He was also still very upset at not being allowed to drive. In his mind any seizures behind the bar would almost certainly reveal his epilepsy, and an innocent inquiry about his lack of a driving licence might one day have the same effect. He more than once intimated that either could occur any day.

Despite his strong sense of felt stigma and of being 'at risk' – a legacy, it seemed, of his mother's reaction to the diagnosis of epilepsy – Ralph could recall *no* occasions on which he had suspected being a victim of enacted stigma, however casual or inconsequential. He had never lost a friend through his epilepsy, and his full disclosure to his 'wife' and her family had led to acceptance rather than rejection. While it could be argued that had he disclosed, or been otherwise discredited, more often in more contexts he might well have suffered from episodes of enacted stigma, there is no doubt *in the event*, either that felt stigma had caused him more anxiety and unease than enacted stigma, or that his experiences were *not* amenable to analysis in terms of the orthodox viewpoint. In both these respects Ralph S. was typical of respondents in Scambler and Hopkins' study.

Alternative forms of adjustment and non-adjustment

West has described an earlier version of the hidden distress model as 'all-embracing' (1986: 250). It appears this way because it purports to represent the most significant or typical mode of coping with epilepsy. There is no denying of course that other strategies may be utilized. West (1985) found that parents of children with epilepsy had three main ways of managing stigma: 'concealing', 'avoidance' and 'avowal of normality'. The strategy of concealing is closest to that epitomized in the hidden distress model. But the hidden distress model may also be said to incorporate the strategy of avoidance: 'Avoidance is closely related to concealing and involves in addition the condoned avoidance of situations outside the family to minimize the risks of misadventure and stigmatization' (1985: 116). Two out of the twenty-four families West studied opted for the very different third strategy involving an avowal of normality. This combined maximum disclosure, to reduce the risk of misadventure, and maximum participation in activities outside the family, to accomplish normal identity. West makes the point that parents who reported episodes of stigmatization tended to be those whose advocated strategies of concealing and avoidance had failed.

Schneider and Conrad (1981) in the US have produced a typology of modes of adaptation to epilepsy. They distinguish first between 'adjusted' and 'unadjusted' adaptations. Individuals defined as adjusted are those 'able to successfully neutralize the actual or perceived negative impact of epilepsy on their lives' (1981: 214). Three sub-types of adjusted adaptation are specified. The first is the 'pragmatic' type. The pragmatist 'minimizes' his or her epilepsy, personally and with regard to others, but does not invariably try to pass or cover. Rather a policy of selective disclosure to those who 'need to know' is pursued, for example, employers, official agencies, close friends and associates. By combining selective disclosure with a scepticism about 'the possibility of others' negative judgements were they to know' the pragmatist effects a relatively normal life.

The second category is the 'secret' type. Epilepsy is managed here by 'sometimes elaborate procedures to control and conceal information about what is perceived as a stigmatizing, negative and "bad" quality of self' (Schneider and Conrad 1981: 215). If successful, this strategy allows cautious participation in most if not all walks of life (including driving, if the individual is willing to lie on application and renewal forms). Third, Schneider and Conrad refer to the 'quasi-liberated' type. Like the pragmatists, individuals in this category straightforwardly acknowledge their epilepsy, but, unlike the pragmatists, they go on to 'broadcast' this information about themselves, both to educate others and to release themselves from any gnawing burdens of concealment based on fear of stigmatization. Drawing on his own experience of coping with psoriasis, Jobling sums up the reasoning behind such a policy of 'de-stigmatization' as follows: 'Deviance is shown to be no more than difference and discredit is denied' (1977: 83).

Unlike adjusted adaptations to epilepsy, which are characterized by a sense of agency or control, the unadjusted adaptation is marked by a sense of being 'overwhelmed' by it. Schneider and Conrad write: 'People who speak of the condition as having a great negative impact on their lives and who seem to have developed no strategies for managing this impact we call "unadjusted" ' (1981: 216–7). They specify one 'extreme' sub-type, which they refer to as the 'debilitated' type. They suggest that this type approximates to what Hughes called a 'master status' that floods one's identity and life with meanings and behaviour that 'figuratively constipate the social self'. Expressed in the words of one of their respondents:

> My only way of dealing with it was to close it up inside me. I really didn't know how to handle it. It was very destructive. It overwhelmed me. My mind was so blocked up with epilepsy and its horrors that I couldn't really relate. It was overpowering.
>
> (1981: 217)

After expounding their typology the authors add the important rider that some people seemed to have adopted different modes of adaptation at different stages of their lives.

Scambler (1984) elaborated on the hidden distress model in the light of Schneider and Conrad's account. First, in his study with Hopkins, non-disclosure or concealment seemed to be the *first-choice* strategy for the great majority of people with epilepsy across their various social roles. Regardless of its efficacy, however, it rarely seemed to bring lasting security or peace of mind owing to the stresses associated with felt stigma. Unlike West, Schneider and Conrad perhaps underestimate these stresses. But if concealment was the preferred or prime strategy, it was not of course the only one. A number of individuals had at one time or another and in one role or another utilized the strategy of the pragmatist; in other words, they had on occasions voluntarily disclosed their epilepsy. Unlike Schneider and Conrad's pragmatists, however, most appeared to regard pragmatism as a back-up or second-choice strategy. They tended to disclose only when their first-choice strategy of concealment seemed likely to fail them or to prove counter-productive. Finally, if there were some – intermittent and typically reluctant – pragmatists in the sample, only 2 per cent seemed to belong to West's category of avowers of normality or Schneider and Conrad's of the quasi-liberated.

Second, in Scambler and Hopkins' study people's epilepsy did not always have high salience for them. Indeed, most people for most of the time felt and acted 'just like everybody else'. Their epilepsy gained high salience for them only when some change in circumstances prompted them to engage with or retreat into their 'special view of the world' based on felt stigma. Under the influence of this 'special view of the world' they were predisposed to certain stereotyped behaviours, namely, depending on whether they were discreditable or discredited, attempts to pass or cover respectively.

Probably the change of circumstances most likely to give epilepsy enhanced salience for an individual was a witnessed seizure which had the potential to expose him or her as 'an epileptic'. Seizure frequency was therefore an important consideration. To emphasize that people's epilepsy typically had high salience for them only intermittently, however, it is worth recording that many seizures were not witnessed by others, and that many of those that were were either not recognized as such or were seen only by those in-the-know (Goffman's 'wise'). Nor were seizures very frequent for many people: only 36 per cent had had a seizure in the month before interview and 31 per cent had not experienced one for two years or more.

Third, people's epilepsy commonly had more salience for them in some roles than in others. Sometimes the deviant status of 'epileptic' contaminated a particular role and its corresponding relationships, affecting people, for example, as wives, mothers, employees and so on. Such contamination rarely seemed to affect the whole range of roles, but rather, at any given time, to be more apparent – and people's epilepsy therefore more salient for them – in some than in others. Often, for example, an individual was content and well supported within his or her family but, because of an increase in seizure frequency, suffering from severe felt stigma in connection with his or her discreditable position at work. From time to time, however, some people admitted to moods of pessimism, even hopelessness, when their epileptic status became a (felt or enacted) master status and they thought themselves 'cursed'. When this occurred they might fairly be described as temporary candidates for Schneider and Conrad's debilitated sub-type of unadjusted adaptation.

Psychological and psychiatric sequelae of epilepsy

In the light of the studies of coping with and adjustment to epilepsy just reviewed, all based on the accounts of sufferers themselves, it might be predicted that both children and adults with epilepsy are likely to experience relatively high rates of psychological and/or psychiatric disorder. This does indeed seem to be the case, although accurate estimates of rates are as yet rare. There are three principal reasons for this lack of convincing data. First, there is no one definition of epilepsy which is universally accepted, so studies vary widely in their criteria for inclusion. Second, many studies have relied on self-administered questionnaires to determine the presence or absence of disorder rather than more accurate methods of assessment utilizing formal interviews. And third, most studies have used hospital or clinic populations to estimate rates of disorder, and this practice tends to produce rates which are acknowledged to be artificially high (Fenwick 1987).

After reviewing the main studies, Fenwick (1987) suggests a prevalence of psychiatric morbidity in people with epilepsy of about one third. What seems incontrovertible is that psychopathology is increased in epileptic populations. Hermann and Whitman (1986) argue that the many factors thought to be causally associated with psychiatric or psychological impairment fall into one of three broad categories. They express these as hypotheses: the 'psycho-social' hypothesis, the 'neuroepilepsy' hypothesis, and the 'medication' hypothesis.

The psycho-social hypothesis seems eminently plausible, as has been indicated already. It states that epilepsy exposes sufferers to multiple stresses which culminate in psychopathology. Hermann and Whitman suggest nine 'high risk' psycho-social factors which, in their view, warrant further research.

The first of these is *fear of seizures*. During the 1980s Mittan and his colleagues have drawn attention to the lack of data on people's fears and misconceptions about their seizures and on possible links between the stresses these induce and psychopathology (Mittan and Locke 1982). Mittan found widespread fears of seizures among a sample of patients in the US. Approximately 70 per cent said they were afraid they might die during the next seizure; 46 per cent said they lived in perpetual dread of seizures; and 35 per cent believed that death from seizures was common.

Two-thirds of the sample were clinically depressed, and Mittan hypothesized a causal connection between fear of seizures and their consequences and anxiety, depression, and other forms of psycho-social impairment. More recently he has reported that people with a relatively high level of fear of death and/or brain damage due to seizures do indeed have substantially increased levels of psychopathology, while those with a relatively low level of fear fall within the normal range of functioning (Mittan 1986).

The second factor identified is *perceived stigma*. Epilepsy continues to be regarded as a stigmatizing condition by many commentators and sufferers alike. And this stigma is often thought to predispose individuals to various forms of psychiatric and psychological disorder. One recent study bears on this claim. Arntson *et al.* (1986) conducted a postal survey of 357 people with epilepsy throughout the US. They found their measure of perceived stigma to be positively and significantly related to perceived helplessness, anxiety, depression and somatic symptoms; and there were negative and significant associations with self-esteem and life satisfaction. They conclude that 'the respondents' perceptions of the stigmatizing effect of epilepsy were significantly associated with indexes of psychological and physiological well-being' (1986: 156); but they prudently add that causality has not yet been established.

Perceived discrimination, particularly in the labour market, is another factor commonly thought to underlie psychiatric and psychological disorder. Despite the wide circulation of this view, however, it does not yet appear to have been subjected to empirical evaluation. The same is almost true of the fourth factor, *adjustment to epilepsy*. It has frequently been noted that people with epilepsy resent their condition and have difficulty coming to terms with it; and it has been asserted that this can lead to various behavioural problems, depression and hostility. There is some circumstantial evidence to support this in the work of Dodrill *et al.* (1980). They presented an intercorrelation matrix of the individual scales of the Washington Psycho-social Seizure Inventory, and this showed a high correlation between the Adjustment to Epilepsy scale and the Emotional Adjustment scale, suggesting a substantial association between poor adjustment and psychopathology.

The fifth factor is *locus of control*. Several commentators have claimed that people with epilepsy, by virtue of their lack of control over their seizures and, possibly, other aspects of their lives, tend to develop a fatalistic attitude, or belief in an external locus of control. There is some evidence that this is indeed the case. Moreover, studies by Matthews and Barabas (1986) and Arntson *et al.* (1986), on children and adults with epilepsy respectively, have found statistically significant associations between an external locus of control and psychopathology.

The relationship between *life events*, especially undesirable ones, and both physical and mental ill health is well known. Individuals with epilepsy are known to be more likely to experience undesirable life events than others, although nobody has yet sought to examine the relationship between life events and psychiatric or psychological disorders in epileptic populations.

The seventh factor is *social support*. The role of social support in the relationship between epilepsy and psychopathology has not yet been researched; but it is known that social support can be protective of mental health and Hermann (1982) found that children with epilepsy have significantly fewer friends, fewer contacts with the friends they do have, and fewer social activities and outlets than healthy children. On these grounds the relevance of social support would seem to warrant empirical consideration.

It is perhaps surprising that *socio-economic status* has been neglected in this context. In their review of the epilepsy/psychopathology literature Hermann and Whitman (1984) found that only five of the sixty-four studies they analyzed considered the possible significance of socio-economic status, and 'none considered it in a substantive manner'. It is known that unemployment and underemployment are more common among people with epilepsy than among others (see Chapter 6), and that either can predispose to psychiatric and psychological disorder.

Finally, there is a case for investigating the influence of *childhood home environment*. Rutter *et al.* (1970) found that disturbed home backgrounds and broken family relationships were important causes of psychiatric morbidity for children with or without epilepsy. They also found that having a child with epilepsy in the family is an important source of stress for parents; one fifth of the mothers of a child with epilepsy had a nervous breakdown. How parents cope has clear implications for the psychological well-being of children with epilepsy (see Chapter 5).

While there is reason, and in some cases prima facie evidence, for taking the role of each of these psycho-social variables seriously in the genesis of psychopathology in individuals with epilepsy, it is evident that little worthwhile research has so far been done. This is not the case with the neuroepilepsy hypothesis. Hermann and Whitman rightly present this as the most prominent of their triad of hypotheses. It reflects the conviction that psychiatric and psychological disorders in epilepsy are largely 'a function of central nervous system dysfunction that is either the cause of, associated with, or the result of the patient's epilepsy' (1986: 6). In an extensive review of the adult epilepsy/psychopathology literature, the same authors found that 79 per cent of the non-demographic variables investigated empirically as potential risk factors could be subsumed under the neuroepilepsy hypothesis. Behind this excessive interest in neuroepilepsy variables lies a characteristic and sometimes uncritical commitment to the biomedical model of disease (Engel 1977).

Hermann and Whitman select eight neuroepilepsy variables which they regard as high risk factors for psychopathology. The first of these is *age at onset*. Early age at onset has been associated with a generally increased risk of psychopathology. The onset of temporal lobe epilepsy before the age of 10 has been linked to increased aggression, before puberty to global hyposexuality, and during puberty to increased risk of psychosis. Not all studies, however, are consistent, especially in relation to aggression and psychosis.

There is some empirical support for the commonsense assumption that poor *seizure control* is associated with poor behavioural adjustment. For example, Kogeorgos *et al.* (1982) discovered an association between 'seizure severity' (of which seizure control was a composite variable) and increased scores on the General Health Questionnaire. Seizure severity in temporal lobe epilepsy has also been associated with psychosis, although the published findings in this area have not always been consistent. For example, some researchers have reported an *inverse* relationship between seizures, especially complex partial or temporal lobe seizures, and psychosis.

The *duration of epilepsy* has often been linked with both psychopathology and intellectual functioning. More specifically, it has been found that the type and total number of seizures experienced over a lifetime are related to cognitive function (for example, Dodrill 1982). There is still disagreement as to whether the duration of temporal lobe epilepsy is associated with psychosis.

The fourth factor is *seizure type*. The putative relationship between temporal lobe epilepsy and psychopathology has excited a lot of attention since the Second World War. The picture is a complex one and the considerable research literature is contradictory, doubtless partly because of problems of methodology. For example, laterality of lesion has become an important focus of interest. Several studies have indicated a possible relationship between left hemisphere temporal lobe epilepsy and schizophrenia-like psychosis, aggression and behavioural change. But there exist rival studies which show none of these relationships.

There appears to be more consistency in the association between *multiple seizure types* and psychiatric and psychologial disorder. Although multiple seizure types has been variably defined, it has been found to be significantly associated with increased scores on measures of depression, aggression and psychosis, and with Minnesota Multiphasic Personality Inventory scale scores and Washington Psychosocial Seizure Inventory scale scores.

Aetiology is the sixth neuroepilepsy factor. People with symptomatic epilepsy have generally been found to be at increased risk compared with people with idiopathic epilepsy. There is some indication that in individuals with temporal lobe epilepsy an enhanced risk of psychosis is associated with a history of pre-natal complications and a less frequent family history of epilepsy. While aetiology is clearly relevant, work so far has tended to concentrate rather narrowly on the relationship between temporal lobe epilepsy and psychosis.

It was first suggested in the 1950s that *type of aura* may be associated with an increased risk of emotional and behavioural dysfunction. There is prima facie evidence that people with temporal lobe epilepsy with complex auras experience more psychopathology than those with simple auras. Jensen and Larsen (1979) have reported psychosis in individuals with temporal lobe epilepsy to be associated with auras consisting of illusions and hallucinations.

The final factor is *neuropsychological status*. Seemingly contradictory results exist in this context too, but since the late 1960s there has been an accumulation of studies indicating that psychopathology, particularly in temporal lobe epilepsy, is associated with deficits in higher cortical functioning. There is some evidence that people with widespread cognitive deficits have an increased risk of psychosis.

Perhaps the most interesting property of the large body of

research on the neuroepilepsy hypothesis is its limited return. The contradictory and confusing results are partly due to the almost intractable methodological problems in this area of study. Nevertheless, Hermann and Whitman write of neuroepilepsy factors: 'our analysis of certain subsets of these variables suggest that they are relatively modest in terms of their overall explanatory power' (1986: 13). It is interesting to speculate on what the return would have been from an equivalent investment in research addressing the psycho-social hypothesis.

The medication hypothesis is also reviewed by Hermann and Whitman and four high-risk variables discussed. The first of these is *polypharmacy*. There is now fairly clear evidence that polypharmacy for epilepsy can affect not only seizure control but also cognitive function, mood, and psychological state. A relationship between the number of anti-convulsant drugs taken and measures of psychopathology has also been reported.

The second factor referred to is the *serum levels of anti-convulsant drugs*. Toxic blood serum levels are known to adversely affect behavioural and cognitive functioning, but it seems that these effects may also be found with serum levels of some drugs within the therapeutic range. Reynolds and Travers (1974) found that, after excluding people with signs of drug toxicity, mental symptoms preceding epilepsy, and/or evidence of gross cerebral lesions, those showing clinical evidence of psychomotor slowing, intellectual deterioration, psychiatric illness, or personality change had significantly lower serum phenytoin and phenobarbital levels than those without such changes. It is important to remember that none of the serum levels of the anti-convulsant drugs were in the toxic range.

Type of medication may also be of significance. There is some indication, for example, that carbamazepine, a drug commonly used for partial (focal) seizures (see Chapter 1), may have psychotropic effects. And phenobarbital is generally thought to be associated with irritability and, especially in children, hyperkinesis.

Folic acid levels are the last medical factor selected by Hermann and Whitman. Certain anti-convulsant drugs can lead to folate depletion in cerebrospinal and serum fluid. Low serum folate levels seem, in turn, to be related to psychiatric problems, including depression, dementia, fatigue, irritability and apathy. An increased risk for behavioural disorder has also been noted, but not all studies have generated consistent results.

The most obvious implication of this sketch of the three main classes of high risk factors is how unhelpful it is to think in terms of simple causal relationships between epilepsy and specific psychiatric and psychological disorders. The deficiencies of this way of thinking can be further illustrated by a brief consideration of two assertions, namely, that there is a recognizable 'epileptic personality', and that epilepsy is associated with a diminished, or diminishing, intellect.

The belief in the existence of an epileptic personality has proved remarkably durable.

> Descriptions of traits specific to the 'epileptic personality' include the adjectives 'pedantic', 'circumstantial', 'religiose', 'egocentric', 'suspicious', 'touchy' and 'quarrelsome'. Speech is slow and perseverative and thought processes stereotyped and concrete. In both thought and emotions, the patients were described as 'adhesive', 'sticky' or 'viscous'.
>
> (Fenton 1983: 162)

There is evidence that a small proportion of those with epilepsy – Pond and Bidwell (1960) put it at 4 per cent in their general practice survey – display many of these traits. But such traits are almost certainly the product of severe and multiple handicaps, both personal and environmental. Scott writes: 'brain damage, childhood deprivation, the chronic effects of long continued anticonvulsant drugs, and difficulties with schooling, employment and accommodation may all contribute' (1978: 423). He adds that prolonged disorders other than epilepsy, for example, rheumatoid arthritis and chronic pain, can of course lead to personality change.

Tizard (1962), who authoritatively concludes that there is no such phenomenon as the epileptic personality, has highlighted the methodological problems involved in assessing personality disorders associated with epilepsy. First, there are selection factors: many studies have concentrated on people with epilepsy living in institutions and the results of these may not generalize to people living in the community. Second, allowance needs to be made for the different types of epilepsy and for the presence or otherwise of brain lesions or damage. The claim made recently by some that there is a temporal lobe syndrome may be premature, but it at least has the virtue of greater specificity and testability. A third problem might be added here, namely, that a way must be found for distinguishing between and evaluating the causal contributions of a wide range of psycho-social, neuroepilepsy and medication factors to the personality attributes of people with epilepsy. In other words, the need in this area of research as in others is for 'integrated' research and model-building.

This last point applies equally to the literature on intellectual functioning. A number of unsubstantiated assertions have been made about epilepsy and intellectual deterioration. However, while individuals with epilepsy who have become institutionalized tend to have lower IQs than the population as a whole, those living in the community have a distribution of intelligence very similar to that of the general population. Where cognitive function is impeded, this may be related to psycho-social, neuroepilepsy and/or medication factors. Consistently with the biomedical orientation within medicine, neuroepilepsy factors have been the most investigated in this connection. It is known, for example, that people with seizures due to brain damage have IQs lower, by an average of approximately 5–10 points, than those with seizures of unknown aetiology (Dodrill, 1981); that the earlier the age of onset of seizures, and the longer the duration of epilepsy, the greater the chance of cognitive impairment; and that people with generalized tonic–clonic seizures tend to show more impairment than those with temporal lobe epilepsy. More detailed work on temporal lobe epilepsy suggests that left-sided temporal lobe lesions may be associated with impairment of verbal reasoning and learning, and right-sided lesions with impairment of discrimination and appreciation of temporal and spatial patterns; but not all studies reflect this pattern (Fenton 1983: 155). There is also some indication that transient impairment of cerebral function can occur in association with brief spike-and-wave discharges in the EEG, even in the absence of a clinical seizure. It has been suggested that such episodes may be a factor in accounting for the reading retardation found by Rutter *et al.* (1970) in as many as 1:5 children in their Isle of Wight study.

Once again it is evident that it makes little sense to assert a simple causal relationship between epilepsy *per se* and intellectual impairment. In fact these paragraphs on the so-called epileptic personality and intellectual impairment, coupled with the outline of those psycho-social, neuroepilepsy and medication factors either probably or possibly predisposing to psychiatric or psychological disorders, invite three comments.

First, it needs to be acknowledged that a diagnosis of epilepsy can refer to such a diverse range of conditions and symptoms that epilepsy *per se* is an unacceptable variable in this area of enquiry. Second, there is no doubt that extant research is too narrowly informed by the biomedical model of disease (i.e. addressing Hermann and Whitman's neuroepilepsy and, to a lesser extent, medication hypotheses, at the expense of the psycho-social hypothesis). The role of psycho-social factors in this area has been grossly under-researched, despite ritualistic acknowledgements of their likely significance. Third, studies need to be conducted which both incorporate, and allow assessments of the *relative* importance of, psycho-social, neuroepilepsy and medication factors in the genesis of psychiatric and psychological disorders. More research should be integrated, and therefore interdisciplinary.

Chapter five

The impact of epilepsy on family life

The family, according to Litman, 'constitutes the most important context within which illness occurs and is resolved' (1974: 495). The account of the impact of epilepsy on family life offered here has twin objectives. The first is to see how families react and seek to come to terms with the onset of seizures and the medical diagnosis of epilepsy. The emphasis here is on the accommodation of stigma. The second is to extend the discussion beyond consideration of stigma to sample some of the ways in which epilepsy and coping strategies can intrude upon day-to-day family activities.

Reactions to the first seizure

Scambler and Hopkins (1986) found that nearly half their respondents had experienced their initial seizure by the age of 20, and nearly one-fifth had done so by their tenth birthday. Some people's recollections of what occurred and of family reactions were therefore somewhat clouded. The point was also made in Chapter 2, however, that the main source of the anxiety and trauma respondents seemed to suffer at onset, affecting four out of every five, was the *reactions of others*, especially witnesses. Witnesses' behaviour often struck sufferers as inexplicable, particularly if they had themselves been unaware that they had had a seizure, or out of all proportion to the severity of the event (for example, summoning an ambulance). Not surprisingly in light of the fact that over half of those who were familiar with the circumstances surrounding their first seizure said it occurred at home, most witnesses to onset came from sufferers' families. Indeed over two-thirds of those whose initial medical consultation was brought about by the actions of someone other than themselves saw a doctor as a result of a family initiative.

From the accounts people were able to give there seemed to be three typical responses to onset on the part of family members. These were *concern*, *bewilderment* and *helplessness*. All are reflected in these two reports from spouses who witnessed onset:

Oh I felt terrible! I didn't know what was happening, you see. Fortunately my son came home right at that particular time, and looked out to get hold of the doctor. . . . It absolutely knocked me out completely. . . . I'd never seen anything like it before, all this contraction of the arms and the fingers, and the face all going, the tongue protruding, and gradually falling into a coma.

I just didn't know what the hell was happening: it was as simple as that! I had never seen anybody have a – whatever it was! I didn't know what to do, quite frankly. And it was, if I remember rightly, about 2.30 in the morning, or something like that, and it was – it was just frightening, that's all I can say, I didn't know what to do. I think that's what frightened me more than anything: I just didn't know what to do, how to cope. I didn't know what I should be doing – whether I should be trying to stop it or, or do something; I just didn't know.

Although in both instances sufferers experienced relatively dramatic *grand mal* seizures, their spouses' concern, bewilderment and sense of helplessness characterized almost all family responses to onset. Concern was a natural and predictable product of family relationships which were generally stable and strong. Nor is it surprising that almost as many parents and spouses were bewildered by events as were concerned. As Taylor has remarked: 'Ignorance must cover poverty of experience as well as poverty of education – seeing seizures is not an everyday experience' (1973: 92). Several people thought they were witnessing a heart attack:

Well, the boys were very frightened; and my husband said he was petrified because he thought I'd had a heart attack, and he didn't think I was going to live. He thought I was going to die, and this was his natural reaction, you know; he was completely shattered.

The majority of family observers were also said to have endured a profound and disquieting sense of helplessness. This was partly a function of bewilderment: they had little or no notion of what they could or should do. But the sense of helplessness was not wholly explicable in terms of bewilderment. Many people *discovered* they could do nothing to help; they could neither intervene to arrest the events of onset nor ease or comfort the sufferer while these took their inexorable course. They had either to watch and wait or to seek help from some third, 'expert' party. In the event, 20 per cent of known family witnesses telephoned for an ambulance.

Family responses to diagnosis

It was suggested in Chapter 2 that most people are extremely upset when first learning of the diagnosis of epilepsy. This is fundamentally because they see epilepsy as stigmatizing, a perception rooted in their partial and idiosyncratic internalizations of lay beliefs, attitudes, and practices concerning people with epilepsy. Little was said, however, about the circumstances in which these beliefs, attitudes, and practices are interpreted and internalized. There is some evidence that the family is the single most important filter and point of access to lay culture, particularly when onset is early (West 1979; Schneider and Conrad 1980). Schneider and Conrad, having asked how individuals with epilepsy construct their 'views of others' perceptions', write:

> Conventional sociological wisdom has emphasized direct disvaluing treatment by others. While this interactive experience is undoubtedly important to study, our data strongly suggest that people with epilepsy also learn such views from significant and supportive others, particularly from parents. Parental training in the stigma of epilepsy is most clear for people who were diagnosed when they were children, but *stigma coaches* were also identified by those who were diagnosed when they were adults.
>
> (1980: 36)

They continue: 'Our data indicate that the more the parents convey a definition of epilepsy as something "bad", and the less willing they are to talk about it with their children, the more likely the child is to see it as something to be concealed' (1980: 36). They give the example of a 34-year-old woman, diagnosed when 14; she described her parents' reactions as follows:

> Complete disbelief. Y'know . . . 'We've never had anything like that in our family.' I can remember that was very plainly said almost like I was something . . . like something was wrong. '*We've* never had anything like that in our family.' They did not believe it. In fact, we went to another doctor. And then it was confirmed. And so I started takin' medicine. We never talked about it again. I just took the medicine. They got it refilled and I took it, and never talked about it ever again.
>
> (Schneider and Conrad 1983: 87)

Scambler and Hopkins tapped similar experiences:

> I don't think my mother ever actually told any of our friends, ever actually put that name [epilepsy] to it. I think she probably always refers to it as a blackout. She has never called it epilepsy.

> I don't think she likes to admit or feel that I am epileptic, especially as it's come down from her family as far as we know. . . . I don't think she likes to admit it to herself that she's got a daughter who's epileptic.

> Well, when the chap from the ambulance went and told my parents, my father nearly punched him on the nose! I think he was very upset; he kept saying: 'No, she doesn't have fits!'

> Mother has always turned her face against it, that they're not fits. You know, she still doesn't believe they're fits.

> Well, my mum and dad didn't tell my sister much in case she went around telling everybody. It's not something they like to speak about. . . . I think they know what's the matter but no one speaks about it.

> Mother wanted to keep it a big, dark secret and not let anyone know. I just didn't speak about it anyway. . . . It was the sort of thing, if something was let slip, you know, she'd say to Jean [a sister]: 'Shhh!'

> Nobody really said 'epilepsy'. It wasn't – there's a stigma

attached to that, I think. Very much so: it's a dirty word. I don't know whether it's the sound of the word: it struck me that maybe it sounds like 'leprosy' to some extent, you know, and people don't use it at all.

I don't think my mother did tell anybody much, because – well, she didn't like to discuss the affair with anybody. . . . Well, I mean, there's a certain amount of pride, or whatever you like to call it, in disclosing these things, isn't there? . . . It's not a thing to be proud of, is it?

(Scambler 1983)

It was apparent that parents often exercised a considerable influence on respondents' perceptions of the 'public image' of epilepsy. Many parents were told of the diagnosis at a time when their children were too young to comprehend it and opted to conceal or suppress it. As some of the quotations above show, however, not all parents were solely concerned with the welfare of their children: some were worried that the stima of epilepsy would 'spread' to embrace themselves or other members of the family. West, whose investigation was directly focused on families of children with epilepsy, writes: 'That the disvalued status not merely attached to the child but implicated other family members was also indicated by a number of parents' (1986: 255). He cites one parent who, unusually, made an explicit reference to her own sense of 'shame': 'People shy away, and they immediately think there's something wrong with the rest of the family because you've got one like that' (West 1986: 255). West links this phenomenon of affiliational or 'courtesy stigma' with a view that all the parents in his study held at some time or other, namely, that epilepsy 'runs in families'. Thus, epilepsy may bring not only a sense of shame to the family, but also a sense of 'blame'.

If in Scambler and Hopkins' study parents constituted the single most important category of stigma coaches, causally responsible for the development, especially in young children, of the 'special view of the world' described in the previous chapter, they were not the only category. Some spouses had a similar influence. It was also apparent, once again in line with the findings of Schneider and Conrad, that 'close associates, friends, and even professionals sometimes suggested concealment as a strategy for dealing with epilepsy, particularly in circumstances where it is believed to be a disqualifying characteristic' (1980: 36–7). A number of people mentioned the role of physicians in this respect: 'The doctor told my mother not to tell any relatives. But me, I was staggered! I said: "Yes, tell them. It's not worth hiding the truth." '

Mr N. was even more specific, unambiguously attributing his first perception of epilepsy as something to be concealed to a statement by his general practitioner:

I suppose it stems from the fact, when I first contracted it [epilepsy], my doctor said to me: 'If you keep it in your mind to let as few people know about this as possible, it will be in your own interests' – namely, job promotion and things like that.

Aspects of coping in the family

Scambler and Hopkins (1988) found that people's concern and bewilderment abated as they came to recognize seizures as transient and mostly harmless, if sometimes dramatic, intrusions. Their sense of helplessness, however, often lingered on (see also Ziegler 1981). In part compensation for this, many parents and spouses cultivated roles as *protectors* and *comforters*. If they were unable either to arrest or to curtail seizures, they could at least try to ensure that the sufferers sustained no injuries. One respondent recalled:

They just made sure that I hadn't been biting my tongue at all, and just to push a pillow away from my face and make sure there's nothing in the way that can harm me at all, so that I can't crack my head or do anything silly; and just leave me to come out of it myself, not interfere at all.

Tenderness and reassurance could also be shown, and, although they were frequently lost on unconscious or disorientated victims, they afforded a measure of relief from the sense of impotence. 'Mum and dad used to go downstairs and get some, a cold flannel and put it on my head – that's about as much as they could do I think.'

Four out of every five people preferred to be in the company of their parents or spouses, or of somebody else in-the-know, when they had a seizure. They felt safe – from preventable injury, misguided attempts to forcibly subdue them, the summoning of ambulances, effusive pity, enacted stigma, and so on – when in the charge of those Goffman (1968: 41) terms 'the wise'. Pearson has given a graphic account of what can happen if no 'wise' person is around when he has a *grand mal* seizure:

I was really having them bad. . . . They were violent. They were mostly violent because I'd come to and find people holding me down, policemen or whatever, and I became violent because I was being pinned down on the ground by people with their knees in my back. I was always ending up in hospitals and police stations. I just think the policemen were totally ignorant of epilepsy. . . . To them it was a drunk going berserk, or whatever.

I literally was really violent. I was violent if I was interfered with; if I was left alone I was okay. The fact that people came near me and touched me in the fit, held me down, twisted my arms and things like that, their knees on my face, my neck, holding me there. I was reacting really violent; I was reacting *to* violence, I felt like I was defending myself because I didn't know why they were doing this to me. I became violent, went berserk, and would then pass out unconscious for five or six hours.

(Sutherland 1981: 86–7)

Most of Scambler and Hopkins' respondents may have preferred to be in the company of the 'wise' when they had seizures, but few wished to be accompanied by them *in case* they had seizures. In fact, family (and especially parental) *over-protection* was the most common source of anger and resentment against family members. This finding is not a new one (Hoare 1987). Arntson *et al.* (1986) sent questionnaires to over 300 adults with epilepsy in the US, and included the question 'What advice would you give to the family and friends of a person with epilepsy?' The replies are summarized in Table 5.1. It can be seen that a third counselled treating the individual with epilepsy 'normally' (without pity) and one in ten warned against over-protection. Research has accumulated since the 1950s indicating not only a high frequency for parental over-protection – for which Ounsted (1955) introduced the neologism 'hyperpaedophilia' – but also its potentially deleterious effects. Behavioural and personality problems in young adults with epilepsy, for example, have been linked to over-protection.

Table 5.1 Answers given to the question: 'What advice would you give to the family and friends of a person with epilepsy?' (n = 319)

Answer	%
Treat the person normally (don't pity the person)	33
Support the person (love and understand)	31
Learn about epilepsy	14
Don't overprotect the person	10
Get good medical care	3
Keep open communication (listen, share feelings)	2
Find a support group	1
Other	6
Total	100

Source: Arntson *et al* 1986

Schneider and Conrad use the phrase 'disabling parental talk' to refer to statements which 'sounded the theme of restrictions and detailed the things a person with epilepsy could not hope or expect to do' (1983: 88). Such statements were as prevalent amongst their sample of eighty adults as in Scambler and Hopkins' study, although most were confined to leisure activities such as swimming and cycling. In his autobiography, former England cricket captain Tony Greig, who had his first epileptic seizure at the age of 14, wrote: 'My family's reaction was primarily one of protection' (1980: 12). He tells how he fought their well-meaning attempts to constrain him:

> maybe I was foolhardy, a stubborn martyr. But I was lucky. I came to no harm by carrying on just the way I had always done. I never had an attack while on a bike, I never passed out while swimming, and gradually my family realized that they would take half my life away if they insisted on chaining me with safety regulations. So they let me do things my way, possibly reluctantly, possibly fearfully – but, thankfully, without disastrous consequences.
>
> (Greig 1980: 13)

Many children are less willing or able to counter the parental urge to over-protect than Tony Greig was. And as Fenton observed, 'parental over-protectiveness in the long term may encourage the development of life-long passive, dependent attitudes and impair the capacity to establish normal peer relationships' (1983: 154). Lerman (1977) provides an account of the 'typical' effects of over-protection and over-indulgence by parents, which, although exaggerated, reflects an established pattern of research findings. Parents generally react to the diagnosis of epilepsy, he asserts, with a mixture of apprehension, shame, anxiety, frustration, and helplessness. This leads to 'an oppressive atmosphere of secrecy and despair' which has an adverse effect on the child. The child is unable to discuss his or her condition openly and soon comes to see it as something undesirable. Stigmatization may be experienced at the hands of schoolmates, friends, and neighbours who are in-the-know. The child often becomes confined to the home and socially isolated. The intricate skills of social relationships are never learned and he or she remains 'insecure, overdependent, emotionally immature', and is 'inept' when adulthood is reached. Such grim long-term consequences may be rarer than Lerman implies, but they certainly do occur (see the case of Sarah R. discussed below).

Secrecy and concealment

Interestingly, West found that parents who tended to over-protect also tended to favour a policy of concealment. He emphasises the point by comparing such parents with those who opted for a policy of selective disclosure:

> In these cases, particularly those committed to openness, informing others about their child's epilepsy was closely linked with the parental aim of maximizing participation in outside activities. It was perceived as a means of reducing the risk of misadventure and creating conditions for keeping the child normal.
>
> (West 1986: 259).

Of the twenty-four families studied by West, he defines six as successful concealers, six as failed concealers and the remainder as adopting a policy of selective disclosure.

Scambler and Hopkins (1988) report that parents frequently functioned as stigma coaches: through advice and example they prompted 'naive' offspring to define and react to epilepsy as a stigma. A number employed what Schneider and Conrad call a 'closed style':

Parents who adopted this style were described as 'shocked', 'embarrassed', 'ashamed' and 'fearful' to learn their child's diagnosis. These reactions spoke volumes of negative moral meaning to their children, even though, ironically, in many cases few words about epilepsy were ever actually spoken.

(1983: 86)

Scambler and Hopkins found that several parents banned the use of the word 'epilepsy' within the home, let alone outside it. Siblings were often kept in the dark: 'Well, my mum and dad didn't tell my sister much in case she went around telling everybody. It's not something they like to speak about. . . . I think they know what's the matter, but no one speaks about it' (Scambler and Hopkins 1988). Only half of those who had siblings living with them at the time of interview reported that they were aware of the diagnosis. Only older siblings who had witnessed a seizure tended to be told.

The pattern was broadly the same for the children of parents with epilepsy, although far fewer children than siblings were said to know of the diagnosis of epilepsy: only 21 per cent of the children were said to know, compared with 50 per cent of the siblings. More importantly, only 50 per cent of those children who were aged 16 or more and who had actually seen a seizure were said to know of the diagnosis, compared with 86 per cent of those siblings who were aged 16 or over and who had witnessed a seizure. This suggests that parents were even more reluctant to communicate a diagnosis of epilepsy within their families when that diagnosis had been applied to one of them than they were when it had been applied to one of their offspring. It may well be that they felt that to tell younger members of the family of the diagnosis would be to risk its dissemination *outside the family*, that young children would be 'unsafe receptacles for the information' (Goffman 1968: 71). As Mr N. put it: 'one person knows and tells another person, and there it is, it's like a bush fire'. In a small study of twelve families Lechtenberg and Akner (1984) report that children who were not informed about a parent's epilepsy tended to feel unhappy and let down when they eventually found out. They conclude: 'Efforts to conceal the problem breed distrust' (1984: 44).

Not surprisingly very few respondents spoke openly or willingly of their epilepsy outside of their families (Scambler 1983). In fact, nine out of every ten said they had rarely disclosed the diagnosis to people who had not thoroughly earned the status of 'close friend': 'I think I told my closest friends, but I didn't go and broadcast it around, if you like; it wasn't something I was particularly proud of.' 'Only the people I really call "friends" know.' Nor were all close friends automatically privy to the secret, even if they had first-hand experience of epilepsy: 'I've got a very close friend – as I say, *very* close, his son has fits – but I've never told him I've had fits.' Normally people's general reluctance to disclose was the product of felt stigma: they feared that erstwhile friends would reject them or drift away. Some, although no more than one in twenty, claimed to have had experience of this: 'I made a lot of friends at work, but once they find out what's wrong they never come and visit you.'

This is what I've found – that whenever I tell anybody that I'm epileptic they don't want to know me at all. I've had friends here: as soon as they know I'm epileptic they don't want to know me at all.

Occasionally, however, an individual baulked at the prospect of eliciting too much sympathy rather than too little:

I don't tell a lot of them. As I said before, they start feeling sorry for you – you know, pitying you; and you, sort of, don't know where the pity ends and the friendship begins . . . you can't distinguish them. I want them to like me as I am, not feel sorry for me, which is entirely different.

Decisions about disclosing were perhaps most difficult in the context of boy- or girlfriends. A choice generally had to be made between what Schneider and Conrad (1980) call 'anticipatory preventive telling' – disclosing in the hope of influencing others' reactions should a seizure occur – and a more or less precarious concealment. It is helpful to distinguish here between 'casual' or non-lasting relationships and 'permanent' or lasting relationships. Casual relationships will be considered first. It was not possible to obtain detailed accounts of *all* such relationships, some of them formed decades before interview. However, it was possible to establish that of those who had had more than one boy- or girlfriend since learning of the diagnosis, 13 per cent had always disclosed their epilepsy, and a further 26 per cent had done so at least once; 61 per cent had never done so (Scambler and Hopkins 1988).

As was the case with friends and acquaintances, the general reluctance to disclose to boy- or girlfriends was primarily due to felt stigma, the potent influence of which was reflected in statements like Mrs M.'s:

> It used to annoy me terribly, the shame of it really. I was so ashamed, very much so. . . . My mother didn't like it [epilepsy] either, and it's obviously rubbed off on me. . . . I wanted desperately to be normal. I didn't want people to say: 'Oh, see how she's an epileptic!' To me it was a terrible time, and I used to suffer a lot, worrying in case I did take one, a fit, with one of the boys. I never felt I could tell any of them anyway.

To disclose, many thought, was to invite the termination of a relationship: 'That's when they, sort of, you know, they take you out once, sort of thing, but you don't see them no more. I've had enough, you know.'

How many people *in the event* lost boy- or girlfriends because of their epilepsy? Of those who had had at least one boy- or girlfriend since onset, only 17 per cent judged their condition to have been *a* – but not necessarily *the* – decisive factor in the ending of a relationship; moreover, it had only happened once to each of them.

Permanent or lasting relationships which culminated in marriage were also considered. Before examining people's policies on disclosing prior to marriage, it is worth drawing attention to the fact that many of those who were single when interviewed, and who had pursued a strict policy of non-disclosure to boy- or girlfriends, nevertheless felt they would disclose fully, usually as a matter of principle, to a future spouse. Miss R., single and aged 23 when interviewed, spoke forthrightly for the majority:

> the only person I'll ever tell, of the opposite sex, that I suffer from seizures, is the man that can accept me as I am now, that will say to me: 'Will you marry me?' Then, if he says that, I won't say yes until he's understood fully, until he's come over to the GP and I've asked the doctor to explain it all to him. Once that's done, and once he's fully aware of what's wrong, or what it's all about – let's put it this way – then I would, if he still wanted me, say yes. But to go out with every Tom, Dick and Harry and to tell them you suffer

from seizures, which has nothing to do with them whatsoever because they just want you for, you know, a bit of a fling, no. I won't tell them: it's got nothing to do with them.

It would, she later stressed, be 'simply unfair' to marry without first disclosing one's epilepsy: 'It's like two people getting married and the man suddenly turning round after they're married and saying: "I'm terribly sorry, you can't have children, I'm sterile!" I'd go and bang him over the head.'

It is of course one thing to anticipate behaving appropriately and another to do so. This may partly explain why only 33 per cent of the marriages that occurred after onset were preceded by a full disclosure incorporating the word 'epilepsy'; and only a further 36 per cent by a partial disclosure involving words like 'seizures', 'attacks', 'dizzy spells', and so on. No disclosure at all was made in 31 per cent of the three dozen marriages. Disclosure was almost certainly influenced by the witnessing of seizures. Three-quarters of those who disclosed the diagnosis had had a seizure in the presence of their future spouses, compared with 54 per cent of those who disclosed only their seizures and, predictably, none of those who maintained an absolute silence. There was no evidence that non-disclosure jeopardized marriages later.

Accepting the role of witnessed seizures in prompting disclosures, it remains the case that many people, especially those who decided in favour of disclosing the diagnosis of epilepsy, shared Miss R.'s conviction that to 'come clean' was, quite apart from any pragmatic considerations, the morally correct thing to do. This might be termed *principled telling*, as opposed to *instrumental telling*. The decision to disclose was rarely taken, however, without a good deal of painful introspection and careful rehearsing. Mrs F. admitted to being highly anxious beforehand, but eventually:

> I just told him straight out about it actually – because my mother and father, they both left it entirely up to me. . . . I thought it was the best thing to tell him because, if I'd had one, he probably wouldn't have known what to do or what it was or anything; and so I just told him about it and told him what to do and that was it.

She said to him: ' "It's entirely up to you how you feel about it, because I know not everyone would be willing to accept that sort of thing." And he said it didn't make any difference, you know.'

Mrs W. disclosed in similar circumstances and gave a detailed and emotional account of her fiancé's response:

> He just sort of went, sat there and put his hands up to his face, lit a cigarette – I think he smoked about twenty cigarettes in half an hour. And I said to him: 'Well, what are we going to do, are we going to. . . ?' And I think in that half hour he must have thought of everything that he wanted to think of because he came over, and he cuddled me, and he said: 'I want to marry you. I don't care what happens.'

She broke down and wept.

The main cause of the apprehension experienced by those like Mrs F. and Mrs W. before and whilst disclosing was once again felt stigma. They were convinced they were gambling with possible or probable lifetime partnerships. Felt stigma was also the highest common denominator of decisions either to disclose the seizures but to hold back the diagnostic label, or to reveal nothing at all. This point is now a familiar one and a single illustrative quotation will suffice. Miss G., who lived with her common-law husband, explained how, prior to their union, she had disclosed her 'funny turns' but shrunk from the open use of the word 'epilepsy', even when directly challenged.

> I didn't use the word 'epileptic', no. He asked me if they were epileptic, and I said: 'I assume so from what they told me from the recordings I had of the brain.' I never say definitely: 'Yes, they are.' I just don't like it. . . . I don't think it's a very nice word to use. People associate with words, don't they? And I associate the word 'epilepsy' with somebody of very low intelligence.

Her partial disclosure seemed not to adversely affect the relationship.

Family conflict caused by epilepsy

Apart from a reference to resentment occasioned by parental over-protection, little has been said about epilepsy's potential to generate or trigger *conflict* between family members. Such conflict, it seems, is not uncommon, although it tends to be short-lived and family unity more or less satisfactorily reconstituted. Scambler and Hopkins report that in their study *no* family relationships were permanently severed as a result of epilepsy. One relationship had, however, been irretrievably soured. Mrs W.'s seizures started when she was 16 years old and, according to her reading of events, she became thereafter 'the family scapegoat'. West (1985) has also reported scapegoating in families with an epileptic child. Mrs W.'s mother was the dominant personality in a family which consisted of her parents, herself and a sister. Her mother refused to interpret her seizures as evidence of illness. Instead she: 'Just put it down that I was lippy to her, to my mother, because I used to stick up for my rights indoors, see what I mean?' Her mother continued to take this line – that Mrs W.'s seizures were 'put on' to make life difficult for her – even when confronted by doctors who unambiguously took issue with her. 'She said: "No, there's nothing wrong with her." ' Things eventually reached a head when Mrs W. started courting and her mother 'chucked me out of the house'. The relationship had not been terminated at the time of interview, but it had been permanently scarred.

When individuals fall victim to chronic conditions which are particularly disabling or stigmatizing their families are frequently thrown into states of confusion or disequilibrium. Indeed, 'chronic illness may modify family dynamics and power, so that both the objectives and strategies of patients and families are, at certain stages of the illness, in conflict with each other' (Anderson and Bury 1988: 8). As Miss R. put it: 'My parents had to come to an understanding, and so did I. They had to find their depth, and so did I. We had to walk around rather blindly at first, learning how to treat each other and what to do.' If families in such circumstances are to survive intact, states of equilibrium have somehow to be restored. As highly focused research studies such as those of Davis (1963) and Voysey (1975) have shown, the homeostatic mechanisms at work are often extremely complex. In the final section of this chapter, two extended case studies are used to illustrate how the unwelcome intrusion of epilepsy into the family circle can lead to tension and conflict between family members, and how in such circumstances family life might be reconstituted (Scambler and Hopkins 1988). The two families were chosen, first, because it was possible to interview independently all the relevant members of both families, and second, because they both afforded opportunities to elaborate on themes introduced above. Otherwise the experiences of the two families were typical.

The first case study concerns Daniel and Clara T.: Daniel, a hospital laboratory technician, had his first seizure in bed in the early hours of the morning; he was then aged 47. 'I just woke up one morning and my wife said: "You've just had a fit and I've called the doctor in." ' Clara, a former nurse, also told Daniel she suspected epilepsy. For his part, Daniel was not convinced that anything had happened at all, let alone that he had had a 'fit': 'It was a good long while before I believed I'd had that first attack. Really and truly, I thought she was making some fuss out of nothing.' Nor of course was he willing to entertain the to him ludicrous notion that he was suffering from epilepsy. When the general practitioner arrived, Clara privately told him of her suspicions but there was no further mention of the word 'epilepsy' to Daniel at this stage. He was, however, referred to a specialist.

Between the general practitioner's home visit and his consultation with the specialist, Daniel – to Clara's chagrin – vacillated between angry denials that anything at all had occurred during that first fateful night and a grudging acceptance that something *must* have occurred for Clara and his general practitioner to respond in the way they did. When in the latter frame of mind he was inclined to the theory that he must have suffered some kind of 'turn' as a reaction to suddenly discontinuing the 'massive doses' of librium he had been taking to relieve anxiety caused by a persistent and embarrassing stammer. Clara rejected this theory as nonsense and they quarrelled about it more than once.

Two or three weeks after onset Daniel visited a local specialist who diagnosed 'an epileptiform attack'. Daniel's response was perhaps predictable:

> I was quite prepared for them to call it 'epileptiform' because it seemed to me that there's an essential difference there. . . . 'Epileptiform' meant to me some sort of fit which wasn't really epileptic, but it had the same effect as the epileptic. . . . It isn't necessarily caused by the same thing.

He added: 'I didn't want to be epileptic.'

Although he was now prepared to admit to Clara that he must have had a turn of some sort, Daniel remained adamant that he did not have epilepsy. Nor had he abandoned his own aetiological theory, despite the fact that the specialist had dismissed it; after all, he reasoned, no alternative theory seemed to be on offer! Clara meanwhile was losing her patience. She neither understood nor sympathized with Daniel's attempts to 'negotiate' a release from the diagnosis of epilepsy: 'She just said it was an epileptic fit, and that I should face it!' Clara explained that she became so frustrated by what she regarded as insufferable intransigence on Daniel's part that their marriage was for a time in jeopardy. Following Ferreira (1963), it might be said that Clara had refused to join Daniel in constructing a 'family myth'.

This friction between Daniel and Clara seemed to be directly attributable to their different reference groups or perspectives. Daniel's perception of epilepsy derived predominantly from the perspective of the *lay* community, as he had internalized it, while Clara's derived almost exclusively from the perspective of the *medical* community, as she had internalized it (and she had of course been a nurse for a number of years). Less abstractly, Daniel saw epilepsy principally as a stigmatizing label and was chiefly concerned to negotiate its removal, while Clara saw epilepsy principally as a symptom of disease and, as such, strictly non-negotiable.

By the time of interview, five years and one further seizure after onset, both Daniel and Clara had mellowed and were willing to admit they had grown more tolerant. Although they still perceived epilepsy differently, a 'truce' – based on genuine affection, a modest degree of reciprocal sympathy and a tacit agreement not to use the word 'epilepsy' in each other's company – had permitted a restoration of a state of family equilibrium. Whether or not such a truce would have been possible had Daniel had more than a single seizure since onset is a moot point. As it was, his epilepsy had largely lost its salience.

The second case study involves the R. family. When she had her first seizure at the age of 13, a decade before interview, Sarah R. was living with her parents and two younger sisters, Ann, then aged 11, and Jennifer, then aged eight. It was a close-knit family unit and Sarah was quickly surrounded by love and attention. Her father, a London taxi driver, was especially concerned: 'My father, being a Piscean, the same as myself, we've got rather the same kind of temperament – I'm a bit better than he is! – he cossetted a bit – well, a bit! – he nearly smothered me.' For all the closeness of their relationship, Sarah soon came to resent her father's over-protectiveness:

> I think, when one's done something wrong, and you know you've done something wrong, and you know that if you didn't have this particular illness you'd get the biggest hiding, you know, created; when you get away with that kind of thing, you definitely know that something's missing.

As she got older her resentment became more acute:

> My father used to bring it [her epilepsy] up to make me know that I needed him. You know, as soon as I had my seizures it was like a ball and chain went round me, and he didn't let go. I wasn't allowed to sleep at my friends' houses, things like this, just in case.

The accuracy of this portrait of an over-protective father was confirmed by each of the other three members of the family. Sarah's mother felt her husband, whom she described as 'emotional' and 'highly strung', had behaved 'really badly' from the time of onset onwards:

> He didn't want to leave her. I mustn't leave her. Somebody had to be around her all the time. I did at first, because I think you panic and you don't know what to do, but as time went by I began to realize that it was no good for Sarah doing what we were doing, to pamper her, and so I had to become the hard one, sort of thing.

This led to occasional 'shouting matches' between Mr and Mrs R., particularly when Sarah wanted to go out on her own. Jennifer explained what typically happened:

> You see, my mum would say: 'Go out Sarah', and she'd chuck her out. . . . But my dad would say: 'What if you have an attack?', or something like this. He doesn't mean to, but he lets his feelings out, which is not very good for Sarah.

Ann told the same story:

> *Ann:* My mum was a bit more practical, and she realized that you've got to look after Sarah more than your own feelings, you know. I can't really explain it, but dad's kind of, very possessive towards Sarah;

he'd rather, sort of, shut her up and protect her, while mum says: 'She's got to learn to live with it' – you know, hope to get married and things like that. I think my dad would prefer her to just sit around, you know, not go out with boys. The word 'swimming', it's terrible! Not allowed to do that! And drinking and smoking and things like that.

GS: Does he actively try to stop her doing things like that?

Ann: Yes. Actually nine-tenths of the rows in this house are because of that. If she goes out, you know, dad says: 'Don't do this. Don't do that.' My mother sort of screams at him to shut up and, you know, sort of says: 'She's 23 years old!'

GS: How does Sarah react?

Ann: She doesn't like being molly-coddled. She gets very, very worked up about it, very emotional.

For his part, Mr R. was well aware of his family's, and especially his wife's, disapproval of his attitude towards Sarah:

I get accused of pampering her . . . but I mean, if you put yourself in my place, and you know the kid stands just a couple of feet from the side of the platform, or she wants to go heights and you've read in a book that she's not supposed to go heights – all I'm trying to do is to make her aware of the thing that she's epileptic. She's got to live with it, but she's also got to safeguard herself from hurting herself. . . . But she [his wife] won't have it. She says I pamper her, I worry too much over her, or stop her from doing this, or I spoiled her, or I made her as she is today, which is not really true.

He seemed unrepentant. He recalled a party to celebrate the new year which Sarah had wanted to attend. Jennifer had already provided an account, entirely consistent with those of her mother, Ann and Sarah herself:

She was going out to this party, and straightaway my dad jumped in and said: 'Going to a party all by yourself? Walking through the streets? What if you happen to have an attack?' It was all coming out, and he shouldn't have said it!

Now my mum was thinking exactly the same thing, but she kept it inside and said: 'You go'.

Mr R. justified his intervention in the following, revealing terms:

She wanted to go into a neighbourhood which I thought was a very rough, frightening neighbourhood where a lot of rape has happened. . . . Being a cab driver, I know all these things. I seen it: I was 25 years on night work and I know what can be done. And I said to her, the trains didn't go exactly where she wanted, she had a long walk, and I was very worried about her. But she upset herself because she said I was trying to put her off. . . . This is my fear, in case she had an epileptic fit, that somebody might pick her up, put her in the cab and, sort of, rape her; and I think this would be a very great big damage for her.

Despite having, on average, only one seizure every nine months or so, Sarah normally stayed at home seven evenings a week, shunning all forms of social intercourse. In fact she went out so rarely, doubtless primarily because of the long-term influence of her father, that when she did venture out she behaved with a manifest lack of maturity. As her mother expressed it: 'She doesn't know how to behave in company; it's a terrible thing to say, but she doesn't.' This 'lack of maturity', according to both Ann and Jennifer, was most apparent in the company of men. Ann explained:

If we're out with a group of fellas she giggles a lot; she acts sort of immature, I suppose that's the best way to put it. . . . When she's out she often becomes very, sort of, boisterous, which puts others off, because she's so kind of restricted and she's so uptight in case she has an attack or something.

Jennifer explained how and why she and Ann were generally apprehensive when accompanying Sarah:

I'd like to say to her: 'Sarah, come out with me', but I can't for the simple reason, because she doesn't go out a lot – the last time she came out with us she was very embarrassing. I don't know whether you've noticed but she's very boisterous, she's sort of overpowering . . . and she'll just say the first thing that comes into her mind . . . it's very embarrassing at the time . . . and I find myself making excuses for her. I feel very guilty afterwards for doing it.

By the time of interview Sarah had largely lost the will to go out and mix with others, especially men, and spent most of her time closeted at home with her parents. Ann was probably right when she portrayed her as a particularly sad victim of felt stigma:

I think she thinks she'll get very serious with a fella, it will be the real thing, you know, and she'll tell him and he'll be off. That's what she's scared of. That's why she won't go out most of the time, in case that happens.

She lived, Ann said, in a substitute world of dreams, constructing daily fantasies in which men were invariably the protagonists. Not surprisingly, on those rare occasions when she did find herself in male company she lacked the social skills to cope.

Everybody in the family held Mr R. responsible for Sarah's unhappy, cramped lifestyle. Mrs R. said:

I honestly think she would have outgrown it by now had she been pushed out on her own a bit more. She's in; she's always in! You know, as a child she's always been among grown-ups: she's never been a child, if you understand!

A state of family equilibrium could only be maintained by means of a conspiracy involving Mrs R., Ann, and Jennifer to coax and cajole Sarah to socialize and to circumvent and – if necessary – 'shout down' Mr R.'s well-intentioned but misguided protests. If Mr R. had mellowed a little over the years, then, as his wife put it: 'I think that's pure perseverance on our part – swearing tactics, you know!'

Chapter six

Epilepsy, work, and disadvantage

In our century work is probably valued more than ever before, and this seems to be true all over the world. . . . Work is valued not only for its instrumental usefulness, that is, as a means to sustenance or financial prosperity, but also for the psychological 'side-effects' which such economic independence gives. It is valued for its 'intrinsic' importance for a person's psychological and moral makeup. Work is thought to play a crucial role in the formation of the core identity, in self-esteem, in overall organization of life, as well as in mental and physical health.

(Safilios–Rothschild 1970: 194)

The opening words of paragraph 142 of the Reid Report on *People with Epilepsy* bear the same message:

For people with epilepsy, as for most of the disabled, useful occupation is of paramount importance. Now that gainful employment is customary for all men, for single and widowed women, and often for married women, it determines the way of life, social and financial status, and the role in society; and it is a source of personal satisfaction, of social companionship, of esteem, of discipline and of purpose.

(CHSC 1969: 41)

These quotations might serve as a 'text' for this chapter.

Research has shown a clear connection between sickness and disability on the one hand, and unemployment, under-employment, and downward mobility on the other. As far as epilepsy is concerned, it has been estimated that there are approximately 200,000 people of working age with epilepsy in the United Kingdom, and that between 50,000 and 100,000 of these may be experiencing moderate or severe problems with employment (Floyd 1986). The present chapter focuses on the prevalence, nature, causes, and impacts of the 'problems with employment'.

Employment status in Scambler and Hopkins' study

Fifty-eight per cent of the respondents in Scambler and Hopkins' (1980) study who were of working age and not engaged in any form of further or higher education were in full-time employment at the time of interview: 74 per cent of the men, 42 per cent of the unmarried women, and 32 per cent of the married women. The equivalent proportions for the general population of Britain at the time were 81 per cent for men, 42 per cent for unmarried women, and 48 per cent for married women.

The social class distributions of those in full-time work, the total sample, and the total household population of England and Wales at the time Scambler and Hopkins' study was undertaken are given in Figure 6.1. In common with most other community studies of epilepsy, these show that the manual or working classes were slightly over-represented in the total sample population. This may be entirely due to an imbalance in the general practice populations from which the sample was drawn. It has sometimes been suggested, however, that the so-called 'theory of social drift' may account for the over-representation of working-class membership in such samples. According to this theory, people who are chronically sick or disabled are unable to maintain their occupational status and drift downwards to lower social-class jobs. There was no evidence in Scambler and Hopkins' study of any significant intragenerational social drift downwards from one social class to another as a result of epilepsy. Of the twenty-five people who were in full-time employment at onset, 28 per cent had been upwardly mobile, 60 per cent had remained in the same social class, and only 12 per cent had been downwardly mobile (see Figure 6.2). Moreover, there was no reason to suspect that any of those who were downwardly mobile owed this to their epilepsy; indeed, they all denied any connection.

There was a small association between social class and employment status. Three-quarters of those who were unemployed were from working-class and a quarter from middle-class households; among those in full-time employment, 64 per cent were from

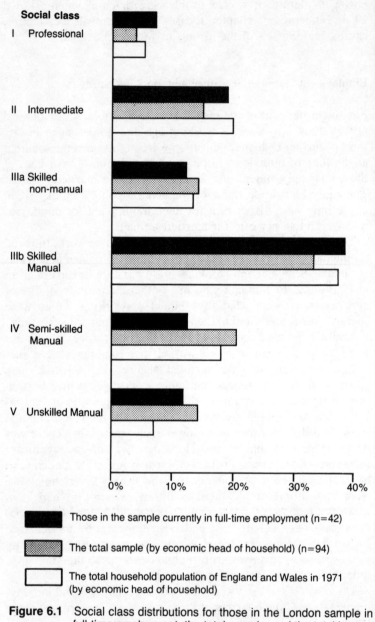

Social class

I   Professional

II   Intermediate

IIIa Skilled
     non-manual

IIIb Skilled
     Manual

IV   Semi-skilled
     Manual

V   Unskilled Manual

0%   10%   20%   30%   40%

Those in the sample currently in full-time employment (n=42)

The total sample (by economic head of household) (n=94)

The total household population of England and Wales in 1971
(by economic head of household)

Figure 6.1   Social class distributions for those in the London sample in
full-time employment, the total sample, and the total household population for England and Wales in 1971

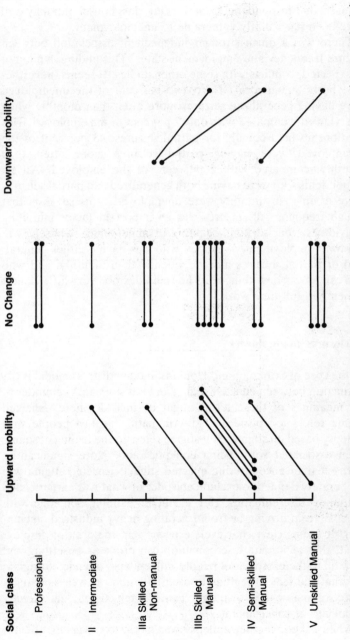

Figure 6.2 Social mobility among those employed at onset. (In each group social class at onset is shown on the left, and social class at the time of interview on the right.) (n = 25)

working-class and 36 per cent from middle-class households. This suggests that respondents from working-class households may well have been particularly vulnerable to unemployment.

There was a much stronger independent association between seizure frequency and employment status. This finding, while not unexpected, conflicts with some other studies. It seems, nevertheless, fairly unequivocal. Thirty-two per cent of the unemployed were having generalized seizures more often than monthly when interviewed, compared with only 2 per cent of the employed. This relationship held equally for partial seizures: 43 per cent of the unemployed were having partial seizures more often than monthly, compared with 7 per cent of the employed. All six respondents who were having both generalized and partial seizures more often than monthly were unemployed. This suggests that a high frequency of seizures was an important factor inhibiting individuals from seeking, securing or maintaining themselves in full-time employment. Anybody who was having either generalized or partial seizures more frequently than monthly, and who also came from a working-class household, stood very little chance of being in full-time work.

Disclosures to employers

At the core of Scambler and Hopkins' hidden distress model is the distinction between enacted stigma and felt stigma. A reminder of the meanings of these terms might be in order here. Enacted stigma refers to episodes of discrimination against people with epilepsy based on stigma. Felt stigma refers to the feeling of shame often associated with 'being epileptic' and, more significantly, to the fear of encountering enacted stigma. Enacted stigma was deliberately defined to exclude episodes of what was earlier called legitimate discrimination (for example, banning someone with epilepsy from driving or from operating heavy industrial machinery). It seems clear, however, especially in the area of employment, that legitimate discrimination can prove as unsettling and harmful to the prospects of people with epilepsy as enacted stigma; and that the fear of legitimate discrimination, as well as being a source of unease in its own right, can, like felt stigma, lead directly to policies of concealment.

When asked whether epilepsy was likely to adversely affect a person's career, all but three of those interviewed felt either that it was or that it could do. Thirty per cent of these were in little doubt:

> I mean, nobody's going to keep a person working for them if they're going to collapse every now and again.

> I can't see them giving you the post if you're an epileptic, rather than John Smith who is perfectly normal.

The other 70 per cent were more circumspect, arguing that whether or not an individual was likely to be a victim of either enacted stigma or legitimate discrimination depended upon any number of factors:

> Well, it all depends on how badly you suffer with it.

> It depends to a certain extent on what type of work you're doing. I mean, if you're coming in contact with the public a lot – well, some people get very nervous, don't they, if they see a person suddenly fall.

> Well, I suppose a lot depends on the employer's attitude. People are still rather inclined to think – if you say 'fits', they rather treat you as a not-very-nice-to-know person.

An individual with epilepsy appears normal between seizures. Goffman has made the point that when a person's stigma is not apparent to others – when a person is 'discreditable' rather than 'discredited' – then

> the issue is not that of managing tension generated during social contacts, but rather that of managing information about his failing. To display or not to display; to tell or not to tell; to let on or not to let on; to lie or not to lie; and in each case, to whom, how, when, and where?
>
> (Goffman 1968: 57)

The temptation for the individual with epilepsy not to disclose to an employer, to attempt to pass as 'normal', is clear:

> I'm nearly certain, if the firm found out that I was having blackouts, they would just take me off the machine, you know, and put me on another job – packing.

> I still feel that there is a certain stigma involved. If I suffered

from, say a weak heart, I don't think I would hesitate to say to anyone I was chatting to that I had a weak heart. But I don't know, you know – for instance, my headmaster, he doesn't know that I'm an epileptic.

I thought perhaps questions may have been asked and I didn't like to, sort of, advertise the fact because I wanted the job, sort of thing. Whether it would have had any bearing I don't know.

Mr W.'s case was an interesting one. He was a 37-year-old executive with a large retailing concern. He explained his policy, consistent with an 'unwritten law' of the company, toward taking on people with epilepsy:

If I'm employing staff and they've got epilepsy, I don't take them on. It's purely business: it's as simple as that. They're there to serve the public and, you know, you certainly couldn't have somebody having a fit behind a counter or in the middle of a store. So, even though I've got a complete understanding of it, I couldn't mix the two, you know, business and my own personal life.

Later he relented a little. If an applicant for a job 'had nocturnal epilepsy, I'd probably take him on. In fact, I would take him on, if he was the right man for the job.' It transpired that Mr W. had convinced himself – unjustifiably as it happened – that his own epilepsy was nocturnal. Nevertheless, it had remained a well-guarded secret. Moreover, he was anticipating a 'medical' at the time of interview, to qualify for a new pension scheme, and fully intended to lie:

I'd lie about it because it doesn't affect my performance. It doesn't affect the company in any way at all because it's nocturnal; and therefore I'm not doing a disservice to the company, or to the insurance company, or to myself, if I don't tell them. Whereas I would be doing a disservice to myself, and to my wife, and to my children, if I did tell them.

He admitted to fearing that he might himself be discriminated against – presumably unfairly – if he did disclose: 'I would think that, if not now, it could be used as a weapon in the future.'

A number of studies have shown that most people with epilepsy are reluctant to disclose to their employers or at job interviews.

A national survey in the US estimated that one third of all people with epilepsy lie about their condition on job applications (National Epilepsy League 1976). In Britain, Jones (1965) found that only 26 per cent of prospective employees with epilepsy at a Welsh steel works admitted their condition at the pre-employment 'medical'. Similarly, Aston found that only 7 per cent of the men at a motor works who were suffering from epilepsy prior to employment admitted as much before starting work (MacIntyre 1976).

Scambler and Hopkins (1980) found that 53 per cent of those who had had two or more full-time jobs after the onset of their seizures had never disclosed their epilepsy to an employer, and only 10 per cent had always disclosed it. As far as those in full-time work when interviewed are concerned, 55 per cent had made no disclosure of any kind to their employers; 17 per cent had mentioned their seizures, often using a more neutral word like 'attacks' or 'turns', but not the diagnosis of epilepsy; and 28 per cent had informed their employers that they suffered from epilepsy. Only one in six made any remarks at all about their condition before being appointed.

Voluntary as opposed to provoked (for example, by a witnessed seizure) disclosure did appear to be associated with seizure frequency: 71 per cent of those who volunteered information to their employers were experiencing more than one generalized and/or partial seizure per annum, compared with only 33 per cent of those who did not. Moreover, more than half those who disclosed voluntarily went on to have a seizure at work, compared with only a quarter of those who did not. Just under a third of those in full-time employment when interviewed had had a seizure at work. Table 6.1 summarizes the data. The figures suggest that respondents tended to be realistic in their attitudes, opting for disclosure when they calculated they were likely to have a seizure at work and against disclosure when they calculated they were not.

Summarizing at this point, it has been argued that because of their fear of encountering either enacted stigma or legitimate discrimination in the labour market people were strongly tempted to keep their epilepsy to themselves. The actual policies on disclosure adopted by respondents in full-time work bore this out: for example, only 17 per cent had disclosed either their seizures or their epilepsy voluntarily, and only 5 per cent had done so before

Table 6.1 Patterns of disclosure among those in full-time employment at the time of interview

Nature of disclosure	%	(cases)	% having a seizure at work	(cases)
No disclosure, or no voluntary disclosure of seizures or epilepsy	83	(33/40)	27	(9/33)
Voluntary disclosure of seizures or epilepsy	17	(7/40)	57	(4/7)
Voluntary disclosure of seizures or epilepsy before starting work	5	(2/40)	100	(2/2)

Source: Scambler and Hopkins (1980)

starting work. Those who did 'choose' to disclose tended to be having more frequent seizures than those who did not; presumably they reasoned that they would probably have a seizure at work sooner rather than later and that an anticipatory disclosure was the lesser of two evils. All this is consonant with the first two of the three propositions constituting the hidden distress model, namely, that when diagnosed as 'epileptic' people develop a 'special view of the world' characterized by felt stigma, and that this 'special view of the world' predisposes them to conceal their epilepsy. It is now appropriate to address the third proposition: that concealment reduces opportunities for enacted stigma, one result of this being that felt stigma tends to be more disruptive of people's lives than enacted stigma.

Discrimination and disadvantage at work

Lennox and Lennox have written: 'The difficulty of continued and satisfactory employment is perhaps the largest practical obstacle that the epileptic has to face' (1960: 950). The work capacity of those who have epilepsy uncomplicated by other problems has been shown to be good (Gloag 1985). Nevertheless, unemployment rates for people with epilepsy are higher than for others both in Europe and the US. American statistics suggest that even those with good seizure control – 75–85 per cent – have a 25 per cent unemployment rate (Holmes and McWilliams 1981), a figure about two and a half times the rate for the population of the US as a whole. Fraser (1980) has argued that if those people with epilepsy who have stopped looking for work are included in the statistics the unemployment rate for all people with epilepsy would be 34 per cent. Nor do unemployment rates provide a full picture. Levels of underemployment are also high (for example, Harrison and Taylor 1976). The findings of a study of an epileptic population in the US by Mittan *et al*. (1983) are fairly typical. Seventeen per cent of white and 43 per cent of urban black patients were unemployed, compared with 8 per cent and 15 per cent of controls coming from the same environment. One-third of the white and one-half of the black group had developed fatalistic attitudes regarding work. Moreover, 71 per cent of those employed expected to lose their job if or when their employers discovered they had epilepsy. British estimates of the proportions of those with epilepsy in the labour market experiencing 'employment problems' vary from between one-quarter and three-quarters. There is no need to review all the relevant studies here, most of which used their own distinctive, and sometimes idiosyncratic, definitions of employment problems. Two studies only will be mentioned, merely to stress the exceptionally important roles of sampling and definitions, namely, those which generated the lowest and the highest estimates of the prevalence of employment problems.

The lowest figure of one-quarter derives from a community survey conducted by the College of General Practitioners (1960). Their figure included the unemployed and all those who fell into a rather vague and heterogeneous category of 'partially employed': 'these were patients whose work had to be modified considerably because of their fits. At home the housewife could only do restricted work; and, outside, sheltered employment was necessary' (1960: 419). The highest figure of three-quarters comes from Jones' (1965) study of applications made by people with epilepsy for jobs at a Welsh steel works. Out of 39 applicants, 33 were appointed. However, over half of those who were appointed subsequently had to change their jobs within the steel works in the face of enacted stigma or legitimate discrimination; these, together with the six rejected applicants, were defined as having employment problems. It must of course be remembered, on the one hand, that Jones' study omitted those individuals with epilepsy who did not apply for jobs at all; but, on the other hand, that it also omitted those who did not disclose their epilepsy to their employer.

Clearly these two studies were conducted with very different populations and utilized very different definitions of employment problems. The material from Scambler and Hopkins' study does not resolve such differences, but rests largely, if not wholly, on respondents' own perceptions of discrimination and disadvantage in employment. For convenience, those who had no experience of full-time work after the onset of their seizures are considered separately and first.

a) people with no experience of full-time work after onset

Seventy per cent of respondents had had at least one full-time job after the onset of their seizures, and 26 per cent had never worked full-time after onset. The remaining 4 per cent were still in educational institutions of one kind or another when interviewed.

It was reported earlier that a higher proportion of women than men were either unemployed or only engaged in part-time work at the time of interview. This expected gender difference was exaggerated for the period between onset and interview: 75 per cent of those who had never been employed full-time after onset were women, compared with only 35 per cent of those who had had at least one full-time job after onset.

Some of the women who had not worked full-time after onset had been too ill to hold down a job. It is reasonable to suggest also, however (especially in view of the fact that four out of every five of them were or had been married), that marriage often functioned to 'protect' women from exposure to the labour market. Because their husbands were normally in receipt of regular salaries or wages, married women often had a realistic option not to work full-time outside the home. Some were doubtless socialized from an early age into taking this option. Others seemed to embrace it through fear of encountering enacted stigma or legitimate discrimination at the hands of prospective employers. In addition, some husbands obviously exhorted their wives not to seek work, either because it was economically unnecessary, or because it was part of their creed that wives should not (have to) work on their own account, or because they too feared the prospect of their wives meeting with enacted stigma or legitimate discrimination – and, consequently, stress and unhappiness – in employment.

Predictably in the light of these remarks, women who married *before* the onset of their seizures were the group most likely never to have worked full-time after onset: they generally enjoyed, or occasionally endured, the 'protection' of their spouses over the entire period from onset to interview. In fact, exactly half of those who had never worked full-time after onset were women who had at some stage been married and who had entered marriage before onset; only 3 per cent of those who had had one or more full-time jobs after onset fell into this same category.

b) *People with experience of full-time work after onset*

It follows from what has been said about those with no experience of full-time employment after onset that those *with* such experience consisted overwhelmingly, first, of men, and second, of women who were either single or who had married *after* onset. These 66 respondents had between them had a total of 249 full-time jobs after onset. Each was closely questioned about his or her work experiences.

Interestingly, although nine out of every ten of these sixty-six people made a general and unsolicited reference to epilepsy as a stigmatizing condition in the course of the interviews, only 23 per cent could recall *a single occasion* on which they *suspected* they had been victims of enacted stigma at their place of work, even of casual and inconsequential teasing.

However, to elaborate on a point made earlier, the experience of enacted stigma in employment is neither a necessary nor a sufficient condition of an inhibited career. It is not a necessary condition because it is possible, for example, for discrimination against a person with epilepsy to have dire consequences for his or her career and yet be fair or legitimate. Consider the recent experience of former world light-welterweight boxing champion, Terry Marsh. Not only was his boxing career instantly terminated by the diagnosis of epilepsy, but shortly afterwards he was 'retired' from his job with the Essex Fire and Rescue Service. Sad though he was, Terry Marsh accepted these actions as constituting legitimate discriminations. And enacted stigma is not a sufficient condition of an inhibited career because it is possible for it to occur without adversely affecting the victim's career (for example, when he or she is merely the butt of an employer's humour).

Forty-two per cent of those with full-time work experience after onset thought their careers had suffered to some extent as a result of either enacted stigma or legitimate discrimination. This compares well with the finding of Ryan *et al.* (1980) in the US that 46 per cent of their sample felt they had encountered employment discrimination due to their epilepsy. Table 6.2 gives details of the types of career inhibitions reported, and of the relative significance of enacted stigma. Thus, for example, 14 per cent felt they had in their time been rejected for one or more jobs because of their epilepsy, and 6 per cent that they had encountered enacted stigma in this context. Similarly, 11 per cent claimed they had been sacked at least once as a result of their epilepsy, and 6 per cent that they had been victims of enacted stigma in being dismissed. In all, 14 per cent felt their careers had been inhibited as a direct result of enacted stigma. There were no associations between the reporting of either enacted stigma or legitimate discrimination and sex, social class, employment status at time of interview, or past maximal frequency of seizures.

Table 6.2 Types of career inhibition due to epilepsy reported by those with experience of full-time employment after onset

Types of career inhibition	People complaining		People complaining of enacted stigma	
	%	(cases)	%	(cases)
Rejected job application	14	(9)	6	(4)
Loss of responsibility or income	12	(8)	3	(2)
Reduced chance of promotion	12	(8)	1	(1)
Dismissal	11	(7)	6	(4)
Withdrawal from work because of pressure by employer	8	(5)	3	(2)
Suspension	3	(2)	1	(1)
Sheltered employment	1	(1)	–	(0)

Source: Scambler and Hopkins (1980)

For all that these estimates of the prevalence of employment discrimination arose out of careful and protracted questioning, it cannot of course be taken for granted that respondents' own judgements of their exposure to such discrimination and of its consequences for their careers were necessarily accurate. The point was made in Chapter 3, in fact, that there is as yet *no* empirical study of discrimination which both uses measures of discrimination which are independent of putative victims' accounts and incorporates comparison groups of people without epilepsy. It needs to be acknowledged, therefore, that the analysis of discrimination offered here remains partial and provisional.

Although the Scambler and Hopkins study did not incorporate a comparison group of individuals without epilepsy, it was possible to compare rates of dismissal from employment *before* and *after* the onset of seizures. Forty-seven people had had a total of 169 full-time jobs before the onset of their seizures, and 6 per cent of these had suffered four sackings. By contrast, 66 people had had 249 full-time jobs after the onset of their seizures, and 27 per cent of these had been the victims of 36 dismissals. Thus, one dismissal occurred in every 40 jobs prior to onset, and one in every seven jobs after onset. These figures suggest that people with epilepsy may indeed be at risk from enacted stigma or legitimate discrimination. However, less than a third of those who had been sacked after onset judged that they had ever been dismissed because of their epilepsy. Post-onset dismissals were not associated with sex or employment status at time of interview. There was no way of telling whether or not they were associated with seizure frequency at the time; given that nearly one-third of those experiencing generalized seizures and one-half of those experiencing partial seizures said their seizures tended to occur in clusters with periods of relative freedom, it is not surprising that there was no association between post-onset dismissals and past maximal frequency of seizures. There was a significant association, however, between residence in a working-class household and being dismissed after onset: over a third of those from working-class households had been sacked once or more after onset, compared with one in ten of those from middle-class households. This reflects the well-documented vulnerability to dismissal of people in manual occupations.

It has been shown that most people with epilepsy concealed their condition whenever possible. Twenty-three per cent of those who had had at least one full-time job after onset had never disclosed their seizures or their epilepsy to an employer. It follows that only 77 per cent had at any time in their post-onset careers afforded employers the opportunity to discriminate against them. This partly accounts for the fact that only 23 per cent reported episodes of enacted stigma at work; and only 14 per cent reported episodes which, in their judgement, had inhibited their careers in some way.

Felt stigma and employment

If the proportion of people in Scambler and Hopkins' study experiencing enacted stigma was not high, many more – nearly nine out of every ten – were made acutely, if intermittently, anxious and unhappy through felt stigma. Most of this distress was occasioned by the perceived need for 'information management': people felt it was in their interests to censor what their employers knew about them. But information management may involve *disclosure* as well as concealment. Schneider and Conrad (1980) have outlined two types of 'instrumental telling' which 'both involve disclosure but, like concealment, are conscious attempts to mitigate the potentially negative impact of epilepsy on one's self and daily round'. They refer to these as 'preventive' and 'therapeutic telling' (1980: 39).

A positive association was revealed earlier between seizure frequency and voluntary disclosure to employers. It was suggested that people who disclosed in these circumstances were often engaging in 'preventive telling'. Schneider and Conrad conjecture that

> to engage in such anticipatory preventive telling is to offer a kind of 'medical disclaimer' intended to influence others' reactions should a seizure occur. By bringing a blameless, beyond-my-control medical interpretation to such potentially discrediting events, people attempt to reduce the risk that more morally disreputable interpretations might be applied by naive others witnessing one's seizures.
>
> (1980: 41)

Preventive telling may also include specific instructions about what witnesses should or – more significantly in view of the lay propensity to summon ambulances – should not do if seizures do occur.

Or therapeutic telling Schneider and Conrad write:

Disclosing feelings of guilt, culpability, and self-derogation can be cathartic. . . . Particularly for those who have concealed what they see as some personal blemish or flaw, such telling can serve a 'therapeutic' function for the self by sharing or diffusing the burden of such information. It can free the energy used to control information for other social activities. Such relief, however, requires a properly receptive audience: that is, listeners who are supportive, encouraging, empathetic, and nonjudgmental.

(1980: 40)

Not surprisingly the authors report this strategy to be most effective with close friends. Scambler and Hopkins' study supported this: while none of those who had worked full-time after onset gave any indication that they had ever disclosed to an employer *primarily* in the hope of some kind of therapeutic return, several undoubtedly did engage in therapeutic telling among carefully selected colleagues or mates.

Scambler and Hopkins found that disclosure to employers seemed rarely to be used as a form of information management. For most, non-disclosure, and not instrumental telling, was the preferred policy. But effective concealment involves more than a decision not to disclose: it involves *not being found out*. It is salutary to recall that three out of every five of those in full-time employment when interviewed who had disclosed their seizures or epilepsy to their employers had only done so under provocation or pressure (i.e. non-voluntarily). Such pressure was usually generated by what might be called 'stigmata' or 'stigma cues'.

Stigmata refer to clinical manifestations of people's conditions, usually seizures, which are noticed by others and which lead to exposure. Mrs G. had a seizure at work and, when she recovered, was asked: 'What's wrong?' She felt compelled to disclose her seizures and the diagnosis of epilepsy: 'Before that I hadn't bothered. You know, I thought. . . . Sometimes people can be catty about things like that. As it happened, they were all very nice about it.' Others were less fortunate. Mrs Z. had a witnessed seizure when filling trays in a factory: 'It was really horrible – all those people staring at you; and you think: "Oh, no! What's going to happen next? Am I going to be sacked?" Or something like that.' Her worst fears were all but realized:

The governor told me he would get my money and my cards ready, but I said: 'No. I don't want to leave. I like it here.' So he said: 'Well, you know you're going to work for less money now, don't you?' And I said: 'Yes, I know.' But in the end I left.

Not all seizures experienced at work are stigmata. Mr N. explained that while he had had seizures at most of his jobs, because these had typically been preceded by an aura he had generally managed to avoid being seen: 'They don't notice it. I just go in the cloak-room – it's empty – and when I'm alright I go back out again.' Even witnessed seizures, especially if they are not *grand mal*, can sometimes be passed off as chance 'faints' or 'turns' (for example, as due to fatigue or the high temperature of the workplace).

It is worth noting that most of those who had disclosed their epilepsy – people, in other words, with no reason to fear exposure through stigmata – nevertheless remained full of trepidation at the possibility or prospect of seizures at work. Goffman refers to the process of 'covering':

It is a fact that persons who are ready to admit possession of a stigma (in many cases because it is known about or immediately apparent) may nonetheless make a great effort to keep the stigma from looming large. The individual's object is to reduce tension, that is, to make it easier for himself and the others to withdraw covert attention from the stigma, and to sustain spontaneous involvement in the official content of the interaction.

(1968: 125)

He adds a little later: 'Many of those who rarely try to pass, routinely try to cover.'

Stigma cues refers to those happenings (excluding clinical mani-festations of people's conditions) which, like stigmata, are noticed by others and ultimately give them away. Examples might include slips of the tongue, overheard conversations, witnessed drug-taking, or absences from work; any of these might function as 'cues' to others, leading them to suspect the victim's 'differentness'.

Consider, for example, absences from work. Pasternak (1981) has recently suggested that, given the competitive ethos of economic life in modern capitalist societies, employers may be reluctant to hire or persevere with people with epilepsy because they perceive them to be less efficient, and therefore as poor investments; and he goes on to mentioned anticipated high absenteeism as one important factor here. It is worth adding at this juncture that a recent study in the British Steel Corporation found no difference between employees with epilepsy and other employees for rates of absenteeism for less than twenty days, although longer absences were more common amongst those with epilepsy (Dasgupta *et al*. 1982; Dick 1986).

Most of Scambler and Hopkins' respondents who had worked full-time after onset and who had disclosed to their employers reported feeling at risk on occasions, or even 'on trial', and were fully aware that any absence from work could – and in some circumstances would – be interpreted as evidence of inefficiency and imprudent or mistaken investment. As a result they often went to great lengths to avoid losing time from work. Mr A. had more than once torn up 'sick notes' signed by his general practitioner because he did not want to (be seen to) take time off, to be (thought) a malingerer. It was with some pride and defiance that he said:

> I could have had an attack last night. How do you know I
> didn't have one during the night? . . . Well, you wouldn't,
> would you? Because, if I'd have had an attack last night, I'd
> have gone to work today and done my job just the same;
> and I'd have been talking to you just normally like I'm talking
> to you now.

Mr N. had an unwitnessed seizure at work and developed a severe headache:

> I was on the verge of going home, but I thought: 'If I go off
> sick, I've got to give a reason'; so I struggled on. And that's
> it. It wore off in the night, you know. It sometimes takes hours
> and hours before your head sort of clears.

When obliged to take time off work, either because of seizures and their sequelae or because of a hospital appointment for example, people frequently attempted to cover; often, they lied.

Of course, for people who had not disclosed to employers, the discreditable rather than the discredited, absences from work were potential stigma cues. They too tended to avoid taking time off if at all possible. Miss C., for example, always arranged for her biannual apppointments at a London teaching hospital to be made during holiday periods. If loss of time was inevitable, people typically attempted to pass; and more often than not, it seemed, passing, like covering, involved prevaricating or lying. Statements like the following were commonplace:

I told them I had the flu.

If I had a seizure in the morning I'd be absent, and if I was well enough I would go in in the afternoon; otherwise I'd go in the next day. . . . I'd tell them I had menstruation pains, which wasn't really a lie because they knew I did.

I think I just said I had a tremendous headache, which was really quite true.

I go to the dentist now when I go to the hospital, don't I?

I just usually said that I wasn't well during the night, you know, and just left it at that, and they've accepted it and haven't asked any more.

The lies and deceit that effective passing sometimes necessitated did not always come easily; often the tension and discomfort of being what Becker (1963) has called a 'secret deviant' was compounded by feelings of guilt associated with the telling of deliberate untruths.

Thus far, support has been adduced for the claim that felt stigma can have a protracted and disquieting effect on people's working lives; but little has been said to buttress the stronger claim that felt stigma is more disruptive of people's careers than enacted stigma. One cannot be dismissed for felt stigma! It can, however, lead directly to career inhibition: people can and do deny themselves opportunities to make or nurture careers through felt stigma.

Mr N. illustrates this. He had been working as a driver for the Post Office for three years before his first seizure. While medical investigations were continuing he took 'a lot of sick leave' and it became necessary for him to see the PO doctor; he disclosed his epilepsy and, as a result, was banned from driving. He immediately and successfully applied for promotion to Postman Higher Grade (PHG), which involved working in the sorting office. About seven years later he noticed a number of vacancies at the London Postal School of Postal Instructors. He sought the advice of his

Head Postmaster, who was in-the-know, not wanting to apply and then be rejected because of his epilepsy. He was told that no 'medical' was involved and that he need not disclose either his seizures or his epilepsy. He applied and was accepted:

> Well, I mean, this was good. This was everything. Everything was flying my way. And then I had an attack. . . . And this happened at the worst time – when I was being trained by another instructor, you see. Well, he must have had some kind of reason: anyway, he told someone, and they told the chief, and I got summoned to the room the next day. And the chief of the Postal School was there, and of course I got the chop.

Mr N. was told that it would be a 'bad influence on other trainees' if he were to have another seizure in front of them. 'So that was finished.' He returned to the sorting office: 'A fallen idol! Not a good thing is it?' He explained what had happened to his Head Postmaster: 'I wasn't going to have it that I wasn't suitable for the job. I'm afraid I couldn't have it that far.' His 'failure' remained a potential stigma cue with regard to his colleagues, however, who knew nothing of his condition. The Head Postmaster was sympathetic. Mr N. himself was bitter. Shortly after, 'following postal reorganisation', he was transferred to another centre, still as a PHG. He was soon recommended by his new supervisor to train as an instructor. He declined, determined not to be disappointed again. In other words, he turned down this second opportunity for career advancement as a consequence of felt stigma: he feared that he would once again fall foul of enacted stigma.

Some married women, with or without coaxing from their husbands, and with varying degrees of insight into their circumstances, clearly opted to forego careers and adopt the 'housewife role' because of felt stigma. Quite apart from any statements by women themselves to this effect, some of the figures cited earlier suggest as much. For example, half of Scambler and Hopkins' respondents who had never worked full-time since the onset of their seizures were married women who had entered marriage before onset. Only 3 per cent of those who had had at least one full-time job after onset fell into this same category. It seems reasonable to argue that felt stigma was probably a key factor in the decisions of married women – who because of their husbands' incomes often had a realistic choice to work in the home rather than outside it – not to forge their own careers.

To summarize, it is well known that people from working-class households are especially vulnerable to employment difficulties; in Scambler and Hopkins' community survey they were more likely to be out of work than their middle-class counterparts. In this context a high rate of epileptic activity can be the straw that breaks the camel's back. Whatever his or her social class, however, someone with epilepsy can be thwarted in the labour market *by his or her epilepsy* only if he or she a) is a victim of enacted stigma, b) is subject to legitimate discrimination, or c) denies himself or herself opportunities by losing the will, with or without justification, to apply for, endure, or advance at work. The third of these may well be as significant as the first and second. Self-denial of opportunities can be understood largely in terms of felt stigma and, to a lesser extent, fear of legitimate discrimination. Felt stigma also predisposes to the concealment of seizures and their diagnostic label from employers. Non-disclosure, in turn, reduces the likelihood of enacted stigma and legitimate discrimination. Felt stigma, quite apart from its role in inhibiting careers, is the prime source of the unhappiness and anxiety that most people with epilepsy intermittently experience at their places of work.

The analyses sustaining these themes have been complex at times. It may be appropriate, therefore, to end this chapter with an additional case study which illustrates several of the chapter's pivotal ideas and concepts.

Miss C. was an infant school teacher in a London school when she had her first *grand mal* seizure at the age of 25. As a consequence of felt stigma she chose not to disclose to her headmistress. She remained discreditable rather than discredited until a few months later, when an absence from work prompted by another seizure functioned as a stigma cue. The headmistress, whom Miss C. had never liked very much, 'seemed sympathetic'; Miss C. felt somewhat ill-at-ease now and again but no kind of discriminatory action was taken against her. Some three years later, however, she had a 'blackout' in her classroom. The noisy, intrigued reaction of her class of infants brought in a colleague from an adjacent classroom, and the pupils were 'shot out while I was dealt with'. Thereafter Miss C. detected a change in the headmistress' attitude: 'she was a bit of a bitch – excuse my language!' Miss C. felt she had become an embarrassment: 'She [i.e. the headmistress] thought that perhaps I'd black out when somone important was being shown round the school. . . . She was that sort of person, you see.' The headmistress also reported the occurrence to County Hall:

> She had to report that I blacked out, and so County Hall sent for me; and I had to be, to have a 'medical'. And of course he . . . said I wasn't fit to teach! We then had fun and games, because my own doctor wouldn't give me a certificate because he said that in his opinion I was perfectly fit and well . . . I think my doctor was quite angry that County Hall had 'suspended' me, because he said: 'There's nothing wrong with you. You're perfectly fit.'

Miss C. remained suspended for an entire term before a decision was anonymously taken that she could return to work. The County Hall doctor told her that had she wanted to *enter* the London area as a teacher she would have been blocked because of her epilepsy; and he added that if she ever moved out of London any subsequent application on her part for a London teaching post 'could be problematic'. Miss C. viewed her 'suspension' and these 'rules and regulations' as forms of institutionalized enacted stigma.

'For some unknown reason' Miss C. went on teaching at the same school for another five years after her suspension. She then resigned in order to take up another teaching post. She disclosed fully to her new headmaster at the time of application, engaging in anticipatory preventive telling, and found him very sympathetic; moreover, 'he kept it to himself'. She had no seizures at work. When the headmaster left four years later, Miss C. took the opportunity to move on to her present post. She opted not to disclose. By this time she was no longer having *grand mal* seizures; in fact, the only clinical manifestations of her epilepsy were periodic bouts of incontinence which she referred to as 'wetting episodes': 'I do have these wetting episodes at school, but you see, I'm so, I cater for myself so well [i.e. wearing sanitary towels] that I usually manage to cope until I can get myself somewhere private to change myself, as it were.' Nevertheless: 'Sometimes I seem to lose every ounce of water within me, and then there's a puddle on the floor.' She continued:

> I try and pretend it hasn't happened. . . . I think one of the

children said once: 'Oh, there's some water on the floor.' And I said: 'and would you like to wipe it up?' And he went and got a cloth and wiped it up; but he didn't connect it with me.

While the discreditable Miss C. professed herself to be 'very happy' in her job, there is no doubt that her wetting episodes could be both deeply embarrassing in their own right and, of course, stigmata. For all that passing had become something of an art, she admitted to walking a tightrope daily; she was a victim of felt stigma.

Chapter seven

Understanding epilepsy better

It has been the aim of this volume to combine highly personal accounts of what it is like to experience epilepsy and all of its psycho-social concomitants with the beginnings of a social scientific analysis of the construction of epileptic identities. To this end there have been fairly detailed considerations of the impact on sufferers of the onset of seizures and the medical diagnosis of epilepsy; of the protracted and often unsettling experience of patienthood; of the tensions and dilemmas faced by their families; and of epilepsy as a potential obstacle in employment. The framework for much of this discussion has been provided by the hidden distress model. This postulates that a deep sense of felt stigma, more often acquired indirectly by coaching than directly by experience, induces a motivation to secrecy which protects from enacted stigma. It is felt stigma rather than enacted stigma which is the principal source of the (hidden) distress of 'being epileptic'.

It is customary in volumes like this to end by calling for additional research. The hidden distress model is clearly embryonic and a number of unresolved issues invite empirical resolution. For example, is the hidden distress model more applicable at some stages in the biographies of individuals with epilepsy than at others? In this connection what, if anything, would a longitudinal study add to the conclusions of the various cross-sectional studies? Not a single social scientific, longitudinal study of epilepsy has yet been published, although analysis of material from the Medical Research Council's National Survey of Health and Development suggests that the hidden distress model may more adequately describe the behaviour of adults than that of children:

Whereas in their school years the children with epilepsy

seemed to have reacted to their illness with some form of aggression and attention seeking, it may be that later in life coping takes a more withdrawn form, anticipated in this study by the greater neuroticism and, later, worse self-perceptions of those who had epilepsy in childhood. At work, this might take the form of an uncomfortable awareness of the need to conceal their illness or its history, . . . and in due course being obliged to take work of a lower social status.

(Britten *et al*. 1986: 242)

The British National General Practice Study of Epilepsy and Epileptic Seizures is an exciting prospective study of patients from the time of their first seizure which, although medically-oriented, will be collecting more psycho-social data in the future; but the study's reliance on questionnaires will impose severe constraints on the kind of psycho-social material obtainable and on its interpretation and analysis.

Probably the most obvious outstanding question in this whole area is: is felt stigma justified? In other words, if people with epilepsy were less secretive, more frank and open in their dealings with families, friends and employers, would the sum total of the unhappiness associated with their epilepsy increase or diminish? Would the prevalence of enacted stigma be significantly greater than it appears to be at present, or not? West has suggested that it might not:

families who have a child with epilepsy can take some comfort from the finding that, in general, those who risked disclosure, and particularly those adopting an open policy, found often to their surprise that the reactions were not as 'negative' as they had expected. The message from this study is that to provide audiences with knowledge in advance of a fit reduces the likelihood of stigmatization; to conceal and encourage avoidance of activities makes both for 'trouble', and increases the likelihood of stigmatization following involuntary disclosure.

(1979: 655)

Rather than trying to resolve issues like these in the absence of telling data, in this final chapter the question will be posed: In the light of what *is* known, what can be done?

What can be done?

There is a clear need for research into the prevalence, causes and principal modes and contexts of enacted stigma in relation to people with epilepsy. It is likely that such research would reveal that enacted stigma is more often an impersonal reaction to the label 'epileptic' than a personal reaction to those unfortunate enough to bear it. Because of the importance of the label, it is worth reflecting on two alternative and contradictory pieces of advice about the future medical diagnosis of epilepsy.

The first prescription, offered sporadically since the 1960s by representatives of the British Epilepsy Association (BEA), is that the diagnosis of epilepsy should be restricted to as few people as possible. Burden, for example, has written:

> We are all endeavouring to avoid talking about the 'epileptic' for two reasons. Firstly, it is well nigh impossible to define what we mean by an epileptic, and secondly, it is socially damaging to be labelled as such. There may be circumstances when you cannot avoid doing so, but I would like to see fewer 'epileptics' if this were possible.
>
> (West 1979: 648–649)

West has countered that this would almost certainly mean that only those with the 'worst' seizures would be labelled 'epileptic'; and this, in turn, would 'merely serve to reinforce the "negative" experience members of the public have, and correspondingly sustain, or even strengthen, "negative" stereotypes' (1979: 649).

The second piece of advice is volunteered by West himself and stands in contradiction to Burden's: it is that more, rather than less, use should be made of the term epilepsy. West suggests, for instance, that it might be desirable to consider febrile convulsions as 'epileptic seizures precipitated by fever', and reports the current estimate that between 5–6 per cent of the population experience at least one febrile convulsion. (He adds, rather cryptically, that defining febrile convulsions as epileptic seizures 'does not necessitate labelling those children as "epileptic" ' (1979: 652).) His thesis, in a sentence, is that extending the use of the term epilepsy should help diminish its associated stigma: 'the range of persons with a history of epilepsy would be increased, and with it perhaps a broadening of experience and commensurate modification of stereotypes' (1979: 653).

It might be objected that both of these well-intentioned pieces of advice are unrealistic and defeatist. They are unrealistic in their shared assumption that both those who experience seizures and members of the public can be duped by an essentially artificial re-definition of epileptic phenomena. And they are defeatist in their seeming acceptance of enacted stigma against people with epilepsy as a *given* in their equations. An alternative, if more mundane, prescription would be to supplement a general improvement in the medical management of epilepsy – which would undoubtedly further reduce the frequency of seizures and hence the problems and dilemmas experienced by sufferers – with a twin assault on poverty of education and, even more importantly, poverty of experience among lay persons.

Judging from the literature reviewed in Chapter 3, it seems that lay persons are better informed about epilepsy than many physicians and others had suspected; it may well be that educational packages deployed by bodies like the BEA have already had some impact, that poverty of education amongst members of the public is being slowly but steadily undermined. Few or no resources, however, have been invested in making good lay poverty of experience. One in three adults has never witnessed an epileptic seizure and, if the medical management of epilepsy is further refined, the proportion of those with even this minimal experience of epilepsy will decrease. It may be worthwhile to prepare lay persons for the experience of *coping* with seizures of all types, perhaps by means of films and simulations. This would not of course lead to the elimination of enacted stigma in relation to epilepsy, but it might conceivably reduce it by removing some of the ambiguity in social interaction caused by the mere presence of an individual with epilepsy. In the long run this may or may not improve the ontological lot of the sufferer.

All this seems far removed from the context in which physician and patient normally meet. What implications do the findings of studies have for routine practice? One of the main sources of dissatisfaction with doctors in Scambler and Hopkins' study was their preoccupation with diagnosis and management and apparent lack of interest in wider aspects of care. The accusation that doctors lack the time, training, or motivation to elicit and address patients' own perspectives on their epilepsy is a common one.

Scambler and Hopkins have distinguished analytically between three common dimensions to patients' perspectives:

a) Felt stigma

In their own study, almost all those interviewed perceived epilepsy as stigmatizing. The term 'felt stigma' was of course coined to refer both to the shame many people experienced and, more especially, to the fear of meeting with avoidance or rejection (i.e. enacted stigma). Felt stigma was the prime constituent of people's perspectives on epilepsy.

b) Rationalization

People are known to be intolerant of uncertainty surrounding illness, particularly if symptoms are serious, dramatic or intrusive. Blaxter (1976) has referred to people's deep need to be able to make sense of what is happening to them. This process of cognitive ordering was earlier termed rationalization.

c) Action strategy

If rationalization is one aspect of adjusting to epilepsy, another is the development of ways of coping with it as a potential personal and social burden. Schneider and Conrad (1981) have suggested that what might be called 'action strategies' can vary between individuals and over time. In Scambler and Hopkins' study, however, the strategy of first choice was concealment: whenever possible people avoided disclosing their symptoms and the diagnosis in an effort to pass as normal.

These dimensions are of course related. In Scambler and Hopkins' study, for example, felt stigma was typically an important factor in rationalization and the key determinant of action strategy.

The evidence from most studies is that physicians tend to be interested in those aspects of patient rationalization that promise to facilitate diagnosis or management, but not in the process of rationalization *per se*. Neither felt stigma nor action strategy tend to be on the medical agenda for consultations, and are typically handled inexpertly and cursorily if raised by patients.

Physicians are often chastised for being poor communicators:

in particular, they are said to impart too little information to their patients. But they can also be poor listeners. In relation to epilepsy it is not enough for physicians to educate patients in the medical perspective, especially if 'compliance' is the sole justification for doing so. It has generally been taken for granted in the relevant literature that patient compliance is a valid measure of medical care. As Mishler points out, 'it requires a shift in perspective and some reflection to recognize that the concept incorporates a medical bias' (1984: 49). It is revealing that although in a number of influential studies a high proportion of patients have reported that physicians did not fulfil their expectations, physicians have not as a consequence been described as 'non-compliant' with patient expectations. Only patients, it seems, are non-compliant.

If this volume has a key message to impart, it is that patients' perspectives on epilepsy need to be respected and explored in their own right. This requires what Schneider and Conrad (1983) have called 'co-participation in care'. As far as the management of epilepsy is concerned, many patients clearly possess relevant expertise and are looking for medical guidance rather than instruction. Consider drug-taking for example. 'Framing the problem as self-regulation rather than compliance allows us to see modifying medication practice as a vehicle for asserting some control over epilepsy' (Conrad 1987). Buchanan (1982) estimates that 75 per cent of his patients show a willingness to assume responsibility for medication. He writes: 'The prime mover in controlling treatment, its dosage and frequency, should ideally be the patient, for it is he who is aware of his seizures, their frequency, and their implications for his lifestyle.'

Beyond management, physicians should encourage the articulation and open discussion of patients' or parents' views on felt stigma, rationalization and action strategy. It may be asking a lot of physicians to suggest that they should evolve comprehensive stigma ideologies or practice theories of the kind envisioned by West, but it is difficult to see how they can provide the kind of counselling increasingly expected of them (DHSS 1986; Oxley *et al*. 1987) unless some progress is made along these lines. Consider, for example, the individual with epilepsy who is trying to work out an action strategy in relation to employment. If his or her doctor is at all responsive, the advice is likely to be to disclose fully and hope for the best. And yet many physicians seem willing to acknowledge that this may be a recipe for disaster. In a recent study of attitudes towards epilepsy in general practice, 78 per cent of those asked agreed that job opportunities for those with epilepsy are restricted. Moreover 88 per cent agreed that employers who claim not to discriminate against people with epilepsy in fact do; only 2 per cent disagreed. And yet, 86 per cent went on to agree that individuals with epilepsy should disclose their epilepsy to prospective employers, with nobody disagreeing (Davies and Scambler 1988). What price help with an action strategy here? Fortunately some attempts are currently being made to clarify medical thinking in this area (Edwards et al. 1986). It is information and open discussion rather than instruction and advice packages that are needed; indeed, open discussion reflective of co-participation in care can be therapeutic in itself.

Mention might finally be made of Anspach's (1979) more radical argument that people like those with epilepsy should focus on the relationships between stigma and society and look to mobilize their resources to forge and present an image of strength to the public. He defines this as 'identity politics' and describes its advocates as 'politicized deviants, collectively engaged in attempts to reweave the fabric of identity'. The aim of identity politics is 'to combat the prevailing imagery' and 'to alter both the self-concepts and societal conceptions of their participants' (1979: 766–7). Dell summarizes:

> Identity politics is not a comforting strategy, either for people with epilepsy or the rest of society, because its demands are equality, not friendship; power, not patronage; assertiveness, not adjustment; politicization of life, not individual despair: the strategy is political rather than therapeutic. Identity politics, as applied to epilepsy, would seek to establish society as the predominant locus of stigma against people with epilepsy. It would demand that the public, when appropriate, view persons with epilepsy as active, viable, strong participants in society who are different because of their seizures but not less than full members of the human race.
>
> (1986: 204)

And, as Anspach maintains, the battle for humanness can itself be health bestowing.

References

Albrecht, G., Walker, V., and Levy, J. (1982) 'Social distance from the stigmatized: a test of two theories', *Social Science and Medicine* 16:1319–27.

Anderson, R. and Bury, M. (1988) *Living with Chronic Illness: The Experience of Patients and their Families*, London: Unwin Hyman.

Anspach, R. (1979) 'From stigma to identity politics: political activism among the physically disabled and former mental patients', *Social Science and Medicine* 13A:765–73.

Arntson, P., Droge, D., Norton, R., and Murray, E. (1986) 'The perceived psychosocial consequences of having epilepsy', in S. Whitman and B. Hermann (eds) *Psychopathology in Epilepsy: Social Dimensions*, Oxford: Oxford University Press.

Awaritefe, A., Longe, A., and Awaritefe, M. (1985) 'Epilepsy and psychosis: a comparison of social attitudes', *Epilepsia* 26:1–9.

Bagley, C. (1971) *The Social Psychology of the Child with Epilepsy*, London: Routledge & Kegan Paul.

Bagley, C. (1972) 'Social prejudice and the adjustment of people with epilepsy', *Epilepsia* 13:33–45.

Becker, H. (1963) *Outsiders: Studies in the Sociology of Deviance*, New York: Free Press.

Blaxter, M. (1976) *The Meaning of Disability: a Sociological study of Impairment*, London: Heinemann.

Britten, N., Wadsworth, M., and Fenwick, P. (1986) 'Sources of stigma following early-life epilepsy: evidence from a national birth cohort study', in S. Whitman and B. Hermann (eds) *Psychopathology in Epilepsy: Social Dimensions*, Oxford: Oxford University Press.

Buchanan, N. (1982) 'Treatment of epilepsy: whose right is it anyway?', *British Medical Journal* 284:173–4.

Canger, R. and Cornaggia, J. (1985) 'Public attitudes toward epilepsy in Italy: results of a survey and comparison with USA and West German data', *Epilepsia* 26/3:221–6.

Carter, J. (1947) 'Children's expressed attitudes toward their epilepsy', *Nervous Child* 6:34–7.

Caveness, W., Merritt, H., and Gallup, G. (1969) 'Trends in public attitudes towards epilepsy over the past twenty years in the United States', in *Exploring World Attitudes Towards Epilepsy*, London: International Bureau for Epilepsy, pp. 5–11.

Central Health Services Council (CHSC) (1969) Advisory Committee on the Health and Welfare of Handicapped Persons, *People with Epilepsy*, London: HMSO.

College of General Practitioners (1960) 'A survey of the epilepsies in general practice', *British Medical Journal* 2:416–22.

Commission on Classification and Terminology of the International League Against Epilepsy (1981) 'Proposal for revised clinical and electroencephalographic classification of epileptic seizures', *Epilepsia* 22:489–501.

Conrad, P. (1987) 'The meaning of medication: another look at compliance', in A. Knopf and H. Schwartz (eds) *Dominant Issues in Medical Sociology*, New York: Random House.

Danesi, M. (1984) 'Patient perspectives on epilepsy in a developing country', *Epilepsia* 25:184–90.

Dasgupta, A., Saunders, M., and Dick, D. (1982) 'Epilepsy in the British Steel Corporation: an evaluation of sickness, accident and work records', *British Journal of Industrial Medicine* 39:145–8.

Davies, D. and Scambler, G. (1988) 'Attitudes towards epilepsy in general practice', *International Journal of Social Psychiatry* 34:5–12.

Davis, F. (1960) 'Uncertainty in medical prognosis: clinical and functional', *American Sociological Review* 66:41–7.

Davis, F. (1963) *Passage Through Crisis: Polio Victims and their Families*, New York: Bobbs-Merrill.

Dell, J. (1986) 'Social dimensions of epilepsy: stigma and response', in S. Whitman and B. Hermann (eds) *Psychopathology in Epilepsy: Social Dimensions*, Oxford: Oxford University Press.

Department of Health and Social Security (DHSS) (1986) *Report of the Working Group on Services for People with Epilepsy*, London: HMSO.

Dick, D. (1986) 'Epilepsy in the British Steel Industry', in F. Edwards, M. Espir, and J. Oxley (eds) *Epilepsy and Employment – A Medical Symposium on Current Problems and Best Practices*, London: Royal Society of Medicine Services Limited.

Dodrill, C. (1981) 'Neuropsychology of epilepsy', in S. Filskov and T. Boll (eds) *Handbook of Clinical Neuropsychology*, New York: John Wiley & Sons.

Dodrill, C. (1982) 'Neuropsychology', in J. Laidlaw and A. Richens (eds) *A Textbook of Epilepsy*, Edinburgh: Churchill Livingstone.

Dodrill, C., Batzel, L., Queisser, H., and Temkin, O. (1980) 'An objective method for the assessment of psychological and social difficulties among epileptics', *Epilepsia* 21:123–35.

Edwards, F., Espir, M., and Oxley, J. (1986) *Epilepsy and Employment – A Medical Symposium on Current Problems and Best Practices*, London: Royal Society of Medicine Services Ltd.

Engel, G. (1977) 'The need for a new medical model: a challenge for biomedicine', *Science* 196 (4286):129–36.

Fenton, G. (1983) 'Epilepsy', in M. Lader (ed) *Handbook of Psychiatry 2: Mental Disorder and Somatic Illness*, Cambridge: Cambridge University Press.

Fenwick, P. (1987) 'Epilepsy and psychiatric disorders', in A. Hopkins (ed) *Epilepsy*, London: Chapman and Hall.

Ferreira, A. (1963) 'Family myth and homeostasis', *Archives of General Psychiatry* 9:457–63.

Floyd, M. (1986) 'A review of published studies on epilepsy and employment', in F. Edwards, M. Espir and J. Oxley (eds) *Epilepsy and Employment – A Medical Symposium on Current Problems and Best Practices*, London: Royal Society of Medicine Services Limited.

Fox, R. (1975) 'Training for uncertainty', in C. Cox and A. Mead (eds) *A Sociology of Medical Practice*, London: Collier–Macmillan.

Fraser, R. (1980) 'Vocational aspects of epilepsy', in B. Hermann (ed) *A Multidisciplinary Handbook of Epilepsy*, Springfield, Ill.: Thomas.

Freidson, E. (1970) *Profession of Medicine: A Study of the Sociology of Applied Knowledge*, New York: Russell Sage Foundation.

Gloag, D. (1985) 'Epilepsy and employment', *British Medical Journal* 291:2–3.

Goffman, E. (1968) *Stigma: Notes on the Management of Spoiled Identity*, Harmondsworth: Penguin.

Goodridge, D. and Shorvon, S. (1983) 'Epileptic seizures in a population of 6000. II: Treatment and prognosis', *British Medical Journal* 287: 645–7.

Greene, G. (1972) *A Sort of a Life*, Harmondsworth: Penguin.

Greig, A. (1980) *My Story*, London: Stanley Paul.

Harrison, R. and Taylor, D. (1976) 'Childhood seizures: a 25-year follow-up; *Lancet* 1:948–51.

Harrison, R. and West, P. (1977) 'Images of a grand mal', *New Society* 40. 762:282.

Harvey, P. and Hopkins, A. (1983) 'Views of British neurologists on epilepsy, driving and the law', *Lancet* 1:401–4.

Hauser, W. (1978) 'Epidemiology of epilepsy', in B. Schoenberg (ed.) 'Neurological epidemiology: principles and clinical applications', *Advances in Neurology* 19:313–38, New York; Raven Press.

Hauser, W. and Kurland, L. (1975) 'The epidemiology of epilepsy in Rochester, Minnesota, 1935 through 1967', *Epilepsia* 16:1–66.

Hauser, W., Anderson, V., Loewenson, R., and McRoberts, S. (1982) 'Seizure recurrence after a first unprovoked seizure', *New England Journal of Medicine* 307:522–8.

Hermann, B. (1982) 'Neuropsychological functioning and psychopathology in children with epilepsy', *Epilepsia* 23:545–54.

Hermann, B. and Whitman, S. (1984) 'Behavioural and personality correlates of epilepsy: a review, methodological critique and conceptual model', *Psychological Bulletin* 95:451–97.

Hermann, B. and Whitman, S. (1986) 'Psychopathology in epilepsy: a multietiologic model', in S. Whitman and B. Hermann (eds)

Psychopathology in Epilepsy: Social Dimensions, Oxford: Oxford University Press.

Hilbourne, J. (1973) 'On disabling the normal: the implications of physical disability for other people', *British Journal of Social Work* 3:497–507.

Hoare, P. (1987) 'Children with epilepsy and their families', *Journal of Child Psychology and Psychiatry* 28:651–5.

Holmes, D. and McWilliams, J. (1981) 'Employers' attitudes toward hiring epileptics', *Journal of Rehabilitation* April/May/June: 20–1.

Hopkins, A. (1981) *Epilepsy: the Facts*, Oxford: Oxford University Press.

Hopkins, A. (1987) 'The causes and precipitation of seizures', in A. Hopkins (ed.) *Epilepsy*, London: Chapman and Hall.

Hopkins, A. and Harvey, P. (1987) 'Epilepsy and driving', in A. Hopkins (ed.) *Epilepsy*, London: Chapman and Hall.

Hopkins, A. and Scambler, G. (1977) 'How doctors deal with epilepsy', *Lancet* 1:183–6.

Hopkins, A. and Scambler, G. (1977a) 'How doctors "manage" epilepsy', in K. Penry (ed.) *Epilepsy: the Eighth International Symposium*, New York: Raven Press.

Janz, D. (1969) 'A comparison of public attitudes towards epilepsy in Germany and the USA', in *Exploring World Attitudes Towards Epilepsy*, London: International Bureau for Epilepsy.

Jensen, I. and Larsen, J. (1979) 'Psychoses in drug resistant temporal lobe epilepsy', *Journal of Neurology, Neurosurgery and Psychiatry* 42:948–54.

Jobling, R. (1977) 'Learning to live with it: an account of a career of chronic dermatological illness and patienthood', in A. Davis and G. Horobin (eds) *Medical Encounters: the Experience of Illness and Treatment*, London: Croom Helm.

Jones, A. (1965) 'Employment of epileptics', *Lancet* 2:486–9.

Jones, A. (1980) 'Medical audit of the care of patients with epilepsy in one group practice', *Journal of the Royal College of General Practitioners* 30:396–400.

Jordan, S., Knight, E., and Vokins, A. (1986) 'Interpreting lay opinions on epilepsy', unpublished pre-clinical project, Middlesex Hospital Medical School, University of London.

Kogeorgos, J., Fonagy, P., and Scott, D. (1982) 'Psychiatric symptom profiles of chronic epileptics attending a neurologic clinic: a controlled investigation', *British Journal of Psychiatry* 140:236–43.

Lechtenberg, R. and Akner, L. (1984) 'Psychologic adaptation of children to epilepsy in a parent', *Epilepsia* 25(1) 40–5.

Lennox, W. and Lennox, M. (1960) *Epilepsy and Related Disorders, Vols 1 and 2*, London: Churchill Livingstone.

Lerman, P. (1977) 'The concept of preventive rehabilitation in childhood epilepsy: a plea against overprotection and overindulgence', in J. Penry (ed) *Epilepsy: the Eighth International Symposium*, New York: Raven Press.

Litman, T. (1974) 'The family as a basic unit in health and medical care: a social–behavioural overview', *Social Science and Medicine* 8:495–517.

MacIntyre, I. (1976) 'Epilepsy and employment', *Community Health* 7:195–204.

Matthews, W. and Barabas, G. (1986) 'Perceptions of control among children with epilepsy', in S. Whitman and B. Hermann (eds) *Psychopathology in Epilepsy: Social Dimensions*, Oxford: Oxford University Press.

Mishler, E. (1984) *The Discourse of Medicine: Dialectics of Medical Interviews*, Norwood, NJ: Ablex.

Mittan, R. (1986) 'Fear of seizures', in S. Whitman and B. Hermann (eds) *Psychopathology in Epilepsy: Social Dimensions*, Oxford: Oxford University Press.

Mittan, R. and Locke, G. (1982) 'Fear of seizures: epilepsy's forgotten problem', *Urban Health* Jan/Feb: 40–1.

Mittan, R., Locke, G., and Gatica, M. (1983) 'Epileptics' attitudes toward finding and maintaining employment', Fifteenth Epilepsy International Symposium, Washington DC.

National Epilepsy League (1976) Personal communication to Peter Conrad.

Ounsted, C. (1955) 'The hyperkinetic syndrome in epileptic children', *Lancet* 2:303–11.

Oxley, J., Espir, M., Shorvon, S., Goodridge, D., and Richens, A. (1987) 'The framework of medical care for epilepsy', *Health Trends* 19:13–17.

Pasternak, J. (1981) 'An analysis of social perceptions of epilepsy: increasing rationalization as seen through the theories of Comte and Weber', *Social Science and Medicine* 15E:223–9.

Pond, D. and Bidwell, B. (1960) 'A survey of epilepsy in fourteen general practices, II Social and psychological aspects', *Epilepsia* 1:285–99.

Pryse-Phillips, W., Jardine, F., and Bursey, F. (1982) 'Compliance with drug therapy by epileptic patients', *Epilepsia* 23:269–74.

Reynolds, E. and Travers, R. (1974) 'Serum anticonvulsant concentrations in epileptic patients with mental symptoms', *British Journal of Psychiatry* 124:440–5.

Rotenberg, M. (1974) 'Self-labelling: a missing link in the "societal reaction" theory of deviance', *Sociological Review* 22:335–54.

Rutter, M., Graham, P., and Yule, W. (1970) *A Neuropsychiatric Study in Childhood*, Philadelphia: Lippincott.

Ryan, R., Kempner, K., and Emlen, A. (1980) 'The stigma of epilepsy as a self-concept', *Epilepsia* 21:433–44.

Safilios–Rothschild, C. (1970) *The Sociology and Social Psychology of Disability and Rehabilitation*, New York: Random House.

Scambler, G. (1983) 'Being epileptic: sociology of a stigmatizing condition', Ph.D. thesis, University of London.

Scambler, G. (1984) 'Perceiving and coping with stigmatizing illness', in R. Fitzpatrick, J. Hinton, S. Newman, G. Scambler, and J. Thompson, (eds) *The Experience of Illness*, London: Tavistock.

Scambler, G. and Hopkins, A. (1980) 'Social class, epileptic activity and disadvantage at work', *Journal of Epidemiology and Community Health* 34:129–33.

Scambler, G. and Hopkins, A. (1986) 'Being epileptic: coming to terms with stigma', *Sociology of Health and Illness* 8:26–43.

Scambler, G. and Hopkins, A. (1988) 'Accommodating epilepsy in families' in R. Anderson and M. Bury (eds) *Living with Chronic Illness: The Experience of Patients and their Families*, London: Allen & Unwin.

Schneider, J. and Conrad, P. (1980) 'In the closet with illness: epilepsy, stigma potential and information control', *Social Problems* 28:32–44.

Schneider, J. and Conrad, P. (1981) 'Medical and sociological typologies: the case of epilepsy', *Social Science and Medicine* 15A:211–9.

Schneider, J. and Conrad, P. (1983) *Having Epilepsy: the Experience and Control of Illness*, Philadelphia: Temple University Press.

Schoenberg, B. (1985) 'Epidemiology of epilepsy', in R. Porter and P. Morselli (eds) *The Epilepsies*, London: Butterworth.

Scott, D. (1978) 'Psychiatric aspects of epilepsy', *British Journal of Psychiatry* 132:417–30.

Scott, R. (1972) 'A proposed framework for analyzing deviance as a property of social order', in R. Scott and J. Douglas (eds) *Theoretical Perspectives on Deviance*, New York: Basic Books.

Stebbins, R. (1970) 'Career: the subjective approach', *Sociological Quarterly* 11:32–49.

Sutherland, A. (1981) *Disabled We Stand*, London: Souvenir Press.

Sutherland, J., Tait, H., and Eadie, M. (1974) *The Epilepsies: Modern Diagnosis and Treatment* (Second Edition), London: Churchill Livingstone.

Tavriger, R. (1966) 'Some parental theories about the causes of epilepsy', *Epilepsia* 7:339–43.

Taylor, D. (1969) 'Some psychiatric aspects of epilepsy', in R. Herrington (ed) *Current Problems in Neuropsychiatry*, Ashford: Headley Bros.

Taylor, D. (1973) 'Aspects of seizure disorders: II on prejudice', *Develop. Med. Child Neurol.* 15:91–4.

Temkin, O. (1945) *The Falling Sickness*, Baltimore: Johns Hopkins Press.

Tizard, B. (1962) 'The personality of epileptics: a discussion of the evidence', *Psychological Bulletin* 59:196–210.

Voysey, M. (1975) *A Constant Burden: the Reconstitution of Family Life*, London: Routledge & Kegan Paul.

West, P. (1979) 'An investigation into the social construction and consequences of the label "epilepsy" ', Ph.D. thesis, University of Bristol.

West, P. (1985) 'Becoming disabled: perspectives on the labelling approach', in U. Gerhardt and M. Wadsworth (eds) *Stress and Stigma: Explanation and Evidence in the Sociology of Crime and Illness*, London: Macmillan.

References

West, P. (1986) 'The social meaning of epilepsy: stigma as a potential explanation for psychopathology in children', in S. Whitman and B. Hermann (eds) *Psychopathology in Epilepsy: Social Dimensions*, Oxford: Oxford University Press.

Ziegler, R. (1981) 'Impairments of control and competence in epileptic children and their families', *Epilepsia* 22:339–46.

Zielinksy, J. (1982) 'Epidemiology', in J. Laidlaw and A. Richens (eds) *A Textbook of Epilepsy*, London: Churchill Livingstone.

Name index

Subject index

Epilepsy

The Experience of Illness

Series Editors: Ray Fitzpatrick and Stanton Newman
